OVERCOME PROCRASTINATION & OVERTHINKING (2 IN 1)

DEVELOP YOUR SELF-DISCIPLINE, MENTAL TOUGHNESS, & HEALTHY LIFELONG MINDFULNESS HABITS TO FULFIL YOUR POTENTIAL & SMASH YOUR GOALS

STEWART HUNTER

DEVON HOUSE PRESS

CONTENTS

Part IV
REACHING YOUR UNLIMITED POTENTIAL

INTRODUCTION

It's something most of us do every day and throughout the day, often without even knowing it. It has roots which reach out across our lives, from the deepest core of our minds and bodies through to the people around us and then even further, to the ends of the Earth and even beyond.

Procrastination and overthinking may not seem like a global pandemic, but in fact that's what they are. People all over the world suffer from these often-debilitating conditions. They cripple otherwise-able men and women. They destroy lives, relationships, and companies. People do it on every level of their lives at almost every minute of the day, and it often leads to mental and physical disease and premature death.

If you're reading this, chances are either procrastination or overthinking (or both) are a problem in your life. So, I hope you don't feel alone, as it's a rare person who doesn't succumb to one or the other (or both). And the same things which inspire those unfortunate practices touch upon so many other facets of life that they cannot be ignored, or they will go on to spread like an infection. Anybody who procrastinates or overthinks has to get a grip on those practices now, there's literally no time to waste.

This book will provide you with everything you need to defeat those twin threats to your very life, those enemies of happiness and success. You will come to understand the sources of the emotions which inspire those behaviors. You'll have time-tested techniques which are clear and easy to understand and to put into practice to end and reverse the cycles which perpetuate procrastination and overthinking. And you'll learn to apply them to other facets of your personal and professional life to make your entire world a better and happier place. You'll master self-discipline, time management, relationships, all by finally coming to master your own inner self. It's well within your power, easier than you could have possibly imagined. All you need is the desire (which you've proven) and the commitment.

But don't let that word scare you off. It's a big part of conquering procrastination and overthinking, as it is a big part of anything you may pursue in life. If you've got the commitment, I've got all the information and applicable exercises you need.

And who am I? I'm Stewart Hunter, one of the proud and privileged writers here at Devon House Press. We are dedicated to sharing all the latest information to those in need of making their lives better. We believe everybody's life can be improved, and that this will elevate others and raise our entire society to a higher bar. We use the latest research technology and the latest research to give our readers the full breadth of understanding and all the tools they need to correct the often-deadly behavior in their lives. We remove the stumbling blocks to your success and happiness. And we're proud and pleased to do it.

Because we believe we're not just changing lives, we're *saving* lives. Not only will these techniques make you a better and happier individual, they will make you a happier partner in relationships, marriages, and families. Not only will they make you a better worker or manager, they will propel you up the ladder to greater successes. If you feel as if you're sliding down that ladder, the exercises in this book will reverse that trend! Not only will you learn things that will improve your health and wellbeing, you will learn things which just might prevent premature death.

I suffered from both procrastination and overthinking for most of my life. I always needed extensions on my tax returns, I was often late with credit card payments, and I paid the price in ruined credit and tax penalties. But I built my way back to a position of respect and considerable reward by using exactly these techniques. At the core of these practices is the *Pomodoro* technique, which we'll discuss in greater detail later in this book. But that system of breaking down one huge task into smaller milestones and using a schedule to keep the smaller milestones progressing toward the completion of the greater task, is key to the writing of this book itself! It's the way books are written, the way movies are produced, the way buildings, roadways, cars, and rockets are built. So, you're looking at proof-positive that these techniques work.

I got it in ahead of my deadline too.

Reading this book and coming to truly understand the concepts and practices cannot help but improve your life. If you take just one thing away from this book (improved self-efficacy, the *Eat the Frog* technique) and really apply it, your life will be improved, no question. Apply just two more (time logging, meditation) and your successes will accumulate faster than you can count them. And I'm certain you'll find that they all work together, that the success of one technique will inspire you to adapt yet another. They're all part of a tapestry of self-improvement techniques that will certainly enrich both your personal and professional life. You will learn to achieve any goal and reach your full potential, even to expand that potential! You'll learn to recognize the things that are holding you back and you'll have the tools to overcome them. You'll beat those life-crippling behaviors; procrastination and overthinking, but the benefits will go way beyond that. As I said, it stretches across the Earth and even beyond.

And it does. Read on and you'll see. Your whole world view is about to change for the better. Your life is on the precipice of great change. It's up to you!

But don't let procrastination separate you from these life-altering and life-saving techniques. Don't overthink it to a point where you make no decision at all. Don't let negative self-talk convince you that it won't work or that you're doomed to a life of failure. Those things have likely robbed you of your joy and success for too long. And it doesn't matter if you're a student, a teacher, or a retiree, you can still turn those negative behaviors around. You can still live your best life and be the best person you can be; better to yourself, better to your friends, better to your company, better to society. But you must do it now! There's a lot to cover and time is running out for us all. Let's face it, time is the one thing nobody can afford to waste.

And the particular problem here is that forestalling action is just the inspiration for the book, for my writing and you reading it. That means you'll have to conquer the very things which plague you in order to conquer the things that plague you. But as you'll quickly realize, it's just a matter of taking that first step to break that downward spiral. Just having this book open in front of you *is* that first step, you've already taken it! Now take the second step and read it.

What's more, this is information you can share with those you know and love. These practices are so widespread, and the remedies so logical and simple and effective, chances are you'll want to share this knowledge with your family and friends and coworkers alike. You might pass this information along to your boss or your superiors. They'll be impressed that you know these techniques and that you know how to use them, you're bound to do more than just make a good impression.

So, what are you waiting for? Just for me to end this introduction, I suppose, so that we can get on with the urgent business of changing your views of yourself and the world around you, improving both, and recreating your world as you never thought it could be. It's as simple as turning the page. So, let's get to it!

I

DIAGNOSING THE ROOT CAUSE

WHAT YOU SHOULD KNOW ABOUT PROCRASTINATION AND OVERTHINKING

YOU'RE NOT ALONE IN THIS

Procrastination is defined as postponing tasks, either knowingly or not. It's derived from the Latin *pro-crastinus*, meaning *belonging to tomorrow*. Of course, there's only so much anybody can accomplish in a day, and some things do have to be left to the next day. But when these things are habitually postponed, it's about more than just time management.

People procrastinate doing different types of things, and they do it all the time whether or not they realize it. Estimates are that roughly 20% of people surveyed consider themselves chronic procrastinators. Getting an extension to file tax returns is a classic example of simply putting off an unpleasant chore. Unfortunately, health care is often the subject of procrastination. But people also postpone plans to write a novel, take a vacation, and other pleasant pursuits.

Why is this? Are our daily lives so busy that we simply cannot make time, or are there other things at play? And though we can't add more hours to the day, we can recognize when we've fallen into a cycle of procrastination and how to get out of it, so that we're making the most of the hours and the days which we do have available to us. The old saying goes, "you only regret the things you didn't do." And the reason most people don't do these things is procrastination and over-thinking.

In our increasingly clamorous society, it's increasingly easy to procrastinate. The internet alone provides countless ways to waste time; from videos on YouTube to chatting with friends on Facebook or posting things to your Instagram or Twitter accounts. Countless cable and streaming channels provide more content than any person could watch in a lifetime. So, it's easy to put things off, altogether too easy.

What's important to remember is that virtually anything in life is more important than a video of a baby panda or a rerun of some TV show. Life is short, and procrastination only robs you of what little time you have. That's why it's so important to recognize this dangerous practice and to learn to control it. It's really quite easy, but it does require a bit of awareness and a clear head about what we're dealing with.

People have a variety of reasons for procrastinating and overthinking. They often set standards that are impossibly high, and therefore, they never try to rise to them. They may convince themselves that it's better not to take a risk and fail, or that everything in their lives should be easy and without challenge. When the challenge arises, the procrastinator my blanche at doing anything at all. Other insecurities, such as fear of personal rejection, may be factors as well.

To better understand what procrastination is, it's helpful to remember what it is not. Resting is not procrastination. Nobody can work non-stop; we all need to recharge our batteries. That's part of a well-balanced life. Similarly, procrastination is not laziness. Lazy people lack the goals or motivation to achieve at all. Procrastination happens when a person wants or needs to accomplish a goal but doesn't manage to get around to doing it. Often this is a question of motivation.

One way to look at procrastination is to examine the concept of motivation. If we're highly motivated, we're more likely to accomplish what we need to and less likely to postpone it. Fines and other criminal liability are great motivators to get those taxes filed, right?

But there are different types of motivation, and some are proved to be less successful than others. Extrinsic motivation, or a reward-based motivation, proves to stimulate less dopamine in the brain and therefore, result in a lesser performance. Goal-based motivation is stronger but may have a tendency to lose its potency after the goal is achieved. Intrinsic motivation has, at its core, an internal vision which carries over from goal to goal, one which expresses the creator's true goals in life. Some people used to say that pressure is a great motivator, but we know now that the stress it creates is almost always counterproductive.

Some people are negatively motivated to procrastinate, a sense of rebellion against having to do unpleasant chores in the first place.

However, one may fall into the habit of procrastination, recognizing the cycle is a good way to break it. Generally, procrastination begins with inaction, then guilt which leads to self-doubt, which leads to a feeling of helplessness. Basically, the protagonist may say of themselves, *"I didn't do it, I should have done it, maybe I can't do it, maybe I can't do anything."* Here we see the danger of overthinking, as mentally fixating on this cycle only makes the cycle stronger. More thinking along these lines only makes the problem worse.

Not a very pleasant or productive way to think, is it? Yet it's quite common and well within your ability to solve. One thing to keep in mind is that the cycle can be broken at any stage by simply doing the thing one didn't do in the first place.

A lot of people overcome procrastination by creating a personal vision, one which creates priorities that will motivate and sharpen focus not just one chore but every chore, as they all serve the overall personal vision in one way or another. To-do lists are also a popular and effective way to organize various chores and ensure they get done. Better habits reduce procrastination as well, and many people keep a habit list to help their development of new, better habits as they replace the old, more distracting habits. A lot of procrastinators set time aside for meetings with themselves, where they consider and reconsider their personal vision and to remain focused on their priorities.

THE CONSEQUENCES OF PROCRASTINATION AND OVERTHINKING

The results of procrastination and overthinking can be far-reaching and detrimental. It's about more than not getting some things done, it's about the long-lasting effects it can have on your life.

We've already considered the waste of time procrastination creates, years that pass unproductively, perhaps decades or even an entire life-time. This causes shame, depression, and the downward spiral only gets worse. This creates life-changing opportunities to be missed, either because of depression, a feeling of helplessness to succeed, or simply lack of preparedness. Procrastination and overthinking are often at the root of all three. Procrastination can also prevent long-term goals from being achieved, as it stymies the sufferer who then cannot take the first crucial steps toward improving their lives and accomplishing their goals. Failure to achieve these goals can have career consequences, as a lack of training or development which prevents certain promotions. That lack of professional success can easily cause depression and decreased self-esteem. This can set the stage for poor decisions and lesser goals instead of smarter, long-term goals. This can be damaging to your reputation, further damaging career prospects, inspiring greater depression, and so on. As we can see, procrastination is a downward spiral.

The concrete examples of procrastination's corrosive effect on anybody's life are plain to see and wise to keep in mind. Procrastinating a visit to the doctor or dentist will almost certainly have adverse effects on your health. Procrastinate paying the utility bills and the utilities will be shut off. Miss the tax deadline and there will be fines and perhaps criminal persecution. Put off work or school assignments and you may be sanctioned with a demotion or a failing grade.

Studies also show that procrastinators are more likely to indulge in dangerous activities like smoking, taking controlled substances, unprotected sex, alcohol abuse, and poor driving habits.

At the same time, there can be some benefits to procrastination and overthinking. Taking a bit more time before doing a chore allows for reflection and consideration and may prevent a rushed and therefore lesser performance. Often, procrastination is really just prioritizing. You might do the easier chores on your to-do list first, putting off the more complex chore until the simpler ones are done. And oftentimes, procrastinating doesn't have any obvious long-term effects when the job does finally get done, even if it was at the last minute. A lot of procrastinators see it as a *no-harm/no foul* situation.

Let's take a closer look at overthinking on its own. If procrastination is the forestalling of a certain action, overthinking is often the cause. Examples of overthinking are quite commonplace, and it's an easy trap to fall into. You might be concentrating so hard on a work project that it keeps you up at night. Or you might be reliving an argument you had with a family member and be unable to get it out of your head. If so, you're probably overthinking.

Remember that thoughts cause emotions, and overthinking can create unwieldy, uncontrollable emotions.

Very often, anxiety is at the core of procrastination and overthinking. Anxiety is the normal reaction to stress, but ongoing anxiety is often a hazardous condition or set of conditions; generalized anxiety disorder, social anxiety, or panic disorder. Nearly 40 million American adults suffer from one type of anxiety disorder or another.

Overthinking can lead to analysis paralysis, wherein you may be spending so much effort considering different choices or scenarios that no initial choice is ever made, and nothing gets done at all.

Overanalyzing something can interfere with discovering the solution. Very often our focus can become so fixed on the problem that we lose sight of it. Taking a walk or taking a shower can sometimes break this cycle, as your focus is turned to something simple and mundane which takes little thought, and your mind is unlocked to re-examine the original problem. Overthinking often interrupts sleep patterns, which in turn can have a variety of detrimental effects on both your physical and mental health. Overthinking may trigger mental illnesses and even suicide!

There are a variety of ways you can combat overthinking, including being mindful of the moment and trying not to live too much in either the past or the future, and to be more forgiving of yourself. There are some things you can't control, after all.

And you're not alone. One University of Michigan study found that 52% of 45- to 55-year-olds overthink, and 73% of adults between the ages of 25 and 35 do as well.

A recent U.K. study showed that certain parts of the human brain are more creative when the cognitive process is quieted. According to the study, overthinking naturally thwarts with quieted, creative brain.

Overthinking also eats up a surprising amount of energy and can leave anyone exhausted and unable to break out of the procrastination cycle. And the stress of overthinking may produce the stress hormone called cortisol. But this hormone can be depleted, causing a sort of mental burnout.

Cortisol can also increase your appetite, which creates a pattern of stress eating. This may cause any number of detrimental conditions and diseases including obesity, diabetes, congestive heart failure, stroke, cancer, and any number of other life-threatening maladies. Weight gain can have psychological effects as well, creating depression, loss of self-esteem, isolation and loneliness, and these only contribute to the cycle of procrastination and overthinking.

A Harvard Medical school conducted a study on the brains of subjects at 60-70-years old and contrasted them to the brains of those 100 years old or even older. The results were that those who died earlier had less of the protein which quiets brain activity. Other studies indicate that this protein, RE1-Silencing Transcription (REST), may protect against Alzheimer's disease. But it can be depleted by overuse, which experts believe may be created, in these cases, by overthinking.

Cortisol and other hormones may elevate blood sugar levels and blood fats called triglycerides. That may lead to a host of maladies, including dizziness, fatigue, accelerated heartrate, headaches, difficulty swallowing, inability to concentrate, dry mouth, muscle tension, irritability, nausea, rapid breathing, nervous energy, twitching, trembling, and sweating.

If these hormones are not properly used by the body, the results may include digestive disorders, short-term memory loss, heart attack, premature coronary artery disease, muscle tension, and suppression of the immune system.

Meditation and exercise are good ways to combat overthinking, as is a worry log, or a diary of things which are worrisome or have to be dealt with, a kind of to-do list for your brain. Experts agree that the act of writing is a way to purge the subjects from your subconscious mind and stop the overthinking cycle. Therapy is often recommended, and a strong network of friends and family for support can often make all the difference.

PROCRASTINATION IS A CYCLE, IT EATS UP YOUR LIFE WITHOUT YOU KNOWING ABOUT IT

We've already taken a brief look at procrastination and overthinking as a cycle, feeding upon itself. Procrastination may begin with inaction which leads to guilt, which then may lead to self-doubt, resulting in a feeling of helplessness.

The cycle may also take on physiological aspects; poorer eating habits may create weight gain which adds to the depression, and that depression may trigger the overthinking which stimulates the brain hormones which motivate overeating.

But the cycle of procrastination and overthinking goes even deeper than that. Very often, procrastination begins with hopefulness and determination *("I'll start early this time")* which turns to pressure after the ensuing inaction *("I've got to get started!")*. Here's where anxiety and paralysis step in, and it only gets worse as the procrastinator enters false hope *("I can still do it!")* and then shame and self-recrimination *("Why can't I do this?")* and then often hopelessness *("I just can't do this!")* or a repeating of the cycle with renewed optimism *("I'll start early next time")*. The next day, it starts all over again.

To break this cycle, simply go to the second step. The first step is the same, hopefulness and determination *("I'll start early this time")*. But replace inaction with action in step two. Make a plan, put a to-do list together *("This is how I'll get this done")*. Then use a bit of discipline to avoid the pull of procrastination, *("Why am I resisting this?")* and then take action, even if it's only one step of the project *("I got this done")*.

Let's think of it another way: The various reasons people have for procrastinating, such as fear of failure or a presumption of ease in life, can be thought of as unhelpful rules or assumptions. Going into a task with such rules only creates disgust for the task, leading to distractions and other procrastination activities. They endure the consequences, such as stress or negative socialization, and then wind up procrastinating again the next time.

But a simple change in those unhelpful rules changes everything. Instead of a sense of entitlement, you might assume that most things worth doing in life are going to be a challenge, that nothing worthwhile is ever truly easy. Instead of fearing failure, tolerate the risk. Failure can be corrected, after all, and a failure to act is the true danger in these cases. Simply acting is a victory to a big degree. Changing those unhelpful rules into helpful rules changes the resulting emotion, which will be pride in the progress instead of disgust in the chore. This means dismissing the distracting, procrastination practices and completing the task at hand. The negative consequences of procrastination, the shame and self-doubt, are replaced by pride in achievement and new confidence to get such things done. That inspires you to get the job done the next time and not procrastinate at all.

Voila, the cycle is broken.

WHY IS IT SO IMPORTANT TO CRUSH OVERTHINKING AND PROCRASTINATION?

We've already taken a look at the consequences of procrastination and overthinking; the social pitfalls, the physical and mental and emotional toll it can take. But let's take a look at the other side of that coin and ask what the benefits come from *not* procrastinating or overthinking.

In the same way that procrastinating and overthinking can severely limit what a person may accomplish over their lifetimes, it's also true that not procrastinating created a far more productive life. You may have no idea the things you're capable of or the successes which could be yours simply by making a few small changes to your outlook and your personal habits. The only way to fully plumb the depths of your potential is to act, and that means breaking the cycle of procrastination and overthinking.

Being more productive impacts more lives than just your own. You become an example to others to act and strive to achieve their own goals, and they go on to inspire others. That's a positive cycle you won't want to break, and it will go on endlessly if you remain productive.

You'll also manage to accomplish something; perhaps something small and private, like creating a piece of jewelry or perhaps something big and far-reaching, like creating a jewelry company.

One accomplishment will lead to another, opportunities create opportunities. But you'll only be able move onto the next project once you've completed the current one. Ergo, finish this and you can move on to the next. It'll be helpful if you don't overthink other projects too. Be in the moment and focus on what you're doing instead of what you did or didn't do in the past, or what you may or may not do in the future.

This way, you'll never find yourself in a mental rut, because your new goals and projects will keep you mentally and physically stimulated. And having more to do will encourage better time management.

Perhaps most importantly, you'll learn to take risks and conquer your fears. Franklin Delano Roosevelt famously said, *"The only thing we have to fear is fear itself,"* and it's a perfect way to think about procrastination and overthinking. Anxiety wells up and creates doubt and fear, preventing us from accomplishing the things we want and need to do. But quell the fear with a measure of acceptance, you'll find the courage to move ahead and do what needs to be done. Goals and dreams will come to life, and you will be free of the downward spirals of procrastination and overthinking.

But no book will solve this problem for you. This guide will help you take these steps on your own, create the life you really want. You see the need for a new and better outlook, and you're taking the first vital step on your journey to a happier life. But there's a way to go and little time to get there, so let's get to work and take a closer look at the effects of environment on procrastination and overthinking. That can make all the difference between wasting any more of your valuable time and achieving everything you've ever wanted to achieve.

YOUR ENVIRONMENT COULD BE DRASTICALLY AFFECTING YOUR PRODUCTIVITY LEVELS WITHOUT YOU REALIZING IT

YOU ARE SHAPED BY THE INFLUENCE OF THE PEOPLE AROUND YOU

The people, places, and things around you can have a powerful influence on you, just as you can have a powerful influence on them. It's worth noting here the difference between influence and control. Control is often a futile effort; so many chaotic things can happen throughout the course of a day, a week, or a month, that we can't possibly control all of it, no matter how hard we try. We often can't even control ourselves!

Influence, on the other hand, happens virtually effortlessly. We generally influence those closest to us more strongly than others, and we're likewise more greatly influenced by those who are closest to us. Think of parenting; children cannot always be controlled, but they are always influenced, and by their parents more than anyone else in the early stages of life. Similarly, a child cannot generally control their parents (this is not always true), although, they can influence them in any number of ways. Friends and peers become a major influence once we begin spending more time with them (in school and in the afternoons and weekends) than we spend with our parents (often restricted to a few hours during dinner, if that).

One of the crucial differences is that influence happens automatically, but control requires incredible effort.

So, in dealing with procrastination and overthinking, know first that the best you're likely to do is influence things, not control them; and in a lot of cases that's a lot easier and more effective.

But because influence happens without a concerted effort, one has to be careful not to inadvertently become a bad influence. This requires a little mental discipline, but it's well worth it for you and those around you.

Our moods can influence others, for example. If someone is riding high and another is feeling low, they're likely to draw each other toward a middle ground. Some people in their feelings, one way or the other, and tend to move less and move others more toward their own state of mind. This can be beneficial when the person is upbeat or positive, but when they're constantly negative the situation can be toxic for the other person.

Further complicating things, a single person may be stronger and more resilient on one day, less so on another. Holidays generally find some people on less-stable ground, for example. So, if you're one of them, and the holidays are coming around, it's wise to be aware of your tendencies so you can better control them. The same goes if you know somebody who endures this so you can avoid them during these vulnerable times.

When somebody is a constantly negative influence, there's little you can do to control their perspective. But you can influence by being a consistently better example and hope to elevate them to your level. This is often no easy task, as it means facing and overcoming your own personal negativity, something we can all be subject to from time to time. But that negativity is something to be conquered anyway, so this is as good a time as any!

Cleansing your psyche and elevating your positive influence is a good way to deal with negative influences, but it won't always be enough, and it takes a fair amount of time.

The effects of negativity, from within or without, can be dangerous and shouldn't simply be tolerated. Studies show that even small amounts of negative brain activity may weaken the immune system and lead to heart attack or stroke. According to Dr. Travis Bradberry, negativity can compromise the effectiveness of the neurons in the hippocampus, the part of the brain which handles memory and reasoning.

So, a lot of people recommend simply cutting such people out of your life. If you can't control or influence them, simply remove them from your environment. A principle of Nichiren Buddhism (the oneness of life and its environment) states roughly that our inner selves are reflected in our environment. When we change our environment, we influence our inner selves. If you cut those toxic people from your life, you cleanse your environment and thus, you cleanse your inner self.

Removing such people from your life will free you up to spend more time with better influences and create a stronger, more nurturing environment.

Find such positive influences in volunteer groups, which will elevate anybody's self-esteem. At work, mentors are always a positive influence despite the negative personalities you are likely to come across in almost any work environment.

If you can't avoid such people, set parameters. Physically distance if you can. A lot of negativity comes from self-pity. Instead of letting a complainer go on and on, ask them what positive steps they intend to take to correct their grievance. Resist engaging them in a debate over their feelings; you'll fail to influence them and only come off as bossy or argumentative. Nobody ever wins an argument.

Instead of asserting your perspectives or desires, which are basically irrelevant to such people, consider addressing them in a series of questions instead: *"How does that make you feel? What do you think you can do to change the circumstance so that you feel differently?"*

Again, consider setting the positivity bar higher, in ways that will influence your environment and yourself. Bring some snacks into work, pay somebody a compliment. That will elevate the positivity of everyone around you and that will help you maintain high positivity in return.

Researchers generally agree that negativity can be contagious. Research at the University of Indiana recently found that the negative opinions of others exert a stronger influence on others than positive opinions. Even those with positive opinions were more easily influenced by those with negative opinions, and discussion only increased the influence of the negative influence on the positive.

Psychologist Shilagh Mirgain, PhD puts it this way: "Happiness isn't just a personal experience, it is actually affected by the individuals around you." One person's negativity, for example, can radiate outward to others in that environment, affecting the entire group.

Mirgain's research also indicates that the happiness of a single individual may have a ripple effect of up to three degrees of separation (us, our friends, then our friends' friends). Mirgain also found that negative emotions have a greater impact than positive, often four to seven times greater.

To combat all this external negativity, consider sharing your feelings with those who are sympathetic (even to yourself if need be), surround yourself with positive people whenever possible, and get plenty of sleep. That'll help you to elevate your own positivity and, therefore, the positivity of the people around you.

All that negative energy can have a direct connection to both procrastination and overthinking. Because research increasingly indicates that procrastination isn't the result of poor time management, but of emotional conflict. In fact, poor time management is often seen as a symptom of an emotional problem, not the problem itself.

Rachel Eddins, a licensed professional counselor and American Coun-seling Association member, puts it this way: "There's not one answer to what procrastination is because [there are] so many things that lead to it." So, the best way to deal with procrastination is to first know what the main contributing factors are. Change those factors, change your environment, and you can change your mental state, better understand and overcome the tendency to procrastinate.

Procrastination is an avoidance strategy (literally), and those can create psychological pain which creates depression, anxiety, and other often debilitating conditions.

In 2007, University of Calgary psychologist Piers Steel described four causes of procrastination in what he calls the procrastination equa-tion. The four causes should sound familiar by now:

Low Self-Efficacy: A person's confidence in being able to accomplish the task. Low self-efficacy contributes greatly to procrastination.
Low Value: The pleasantness of the task. Even boring or mildly painful tasks are lower value than extremely difficult tasks.
Impulsiveness: Ability to remain focused and resist distractions.
Delay: How much time until the task needs to be accom-plished. The greater the delay, the more likely one is to put things off.

Steel combines these four elements into an equation which helps anybody calculate how likely they are to procrastinate, and it looks something like this:

Odds of Overcoming Procrastination = Self-Efficacy x Value / Impulsiveness x Delay

So, our self-confidence and the value of the task is divided by one's impulsiveness and the amount of delay. It's tricky, but it can help almost anyone figure out where they fall in the equation. Is self-efficacy the reason for your particular practice of procrastination? Increase it. Too impulsive? Decrease that according to the amount of delay you've got, and the equation should work out.

Here are some specific ways to deal with each of the four:

1. If self-efficacy is the cause, consider breaking the task down to smaller, more manageable blocks to create a series of small victories on your way to completion. That should boost your confidence and reassure you that you can get the job done.

2. If low value is the problem, find a way to increase the value. Make the boring task more pleasant by changing your environment, take your laptop to a public park or café and make it more of an enjoyable task, increasing its value.

3. If you're impulsive, remove those distractions. Turn off the internet, put your phone away, remove anything which distracts you. But don't feel badly about this, as research indicates that the human brain actually requires periodic distractions, it's programmed to work that way. Think about how a small animal will periodically check for danger in its

surroundings, no matter what the animal is doing; eating, drinking, cleaning itself. It's a survival impulse, and it's hardwired into the mammal brain.

4. If delay is your problem, create a series of mini deadlines, think of them as milestones. Time itself will help get the job done.

But outside the famous equation, there are other contributing factors to procrastination, and that brings us back to the environment. Because some procrastination is learned behavior, inherited from those closest to us and thus must likely to have the greatest influence on us. Perhaps a parent or boss or friend or coworker has the tendency, and this influence has affected your behavior too. You won't be able to do much for this person, but you can remind yourself that you can make your own decisions, and that not all influences are positive influences. Use some discipline to be a better influence on yourself.

Another word about controlling your environment before it controls you. The term *priming* refers to the concept of triggers. Walking past Starbucks may trigger your desire for a creamy, high calorie treat. Or walking past the gym may trigger your desire to work out and be healthier. And you can choose to walk past the gym instead of Starbucks if you change your route. Control the triggers in your environment and you can better control your triggers and the desires they inspire. This goes for smartphones, email notifications, and so on.

If you really want to defeat these little distractions, try temptation bundling. Instead of being low value tasks, consider how they relate to your long-term goals. That will make them high value tasks and they will be instantly be more enjoyable. Instead of dreading collecting your bank records for your accountant, think about how much money you'll save on your return this year. Instead of postponing mowing the lawn because of the drudgery of the task, think about how nice freshly cut grass smells, and how good your lawn will look

Rewarding yourself for little victories is another good way to keep yourself motivated. Did you collect and submit your bank records? Have a piece of cake! Mowed the lawn, did you? Sit back and enjoy the ball game! This series of rewards not only reinforces your sense of self-worth and accomplishment but it also gives you incentive to do the less-pleasant chores to begin with. It's what we call a win/win!

DON'T LET TOO MUCH PRESSURE DRAG YOU DOWN

Procrastination and overthinking, by you or someone you are close to, creates pressure. Lost time means harder work which needs to be done faster and, therefore, better. And while some people claim to work better under pressure, they're not taking into account the fact that there are different types of pressure stress. Athletes and artists may endure pressure stress, but this only helps them focus. The stress may even help the overall outcome. In this kind of stress, the person is fixed on the performance and that stress often creates transcendent results.

Destructive stress puts the focus on the person, not the task, and generally produces far lesser results. Destructive stress often results in mistakes. So, know what kind of pressure you're facing and which to avoid.

The pressure of procrastination and overthinking can come from inside and from outside. Other people's opinions, criticism, rejection, the external pressures often foster the tendency to overthink and procrastinate, as we've already discussed. Negative thinking around you can also be a real source of external pressure. But you can use that as motivation to do better, succeed, and be promoted to a better environment. The way you deal with overthinkers and procrastinators will determine how well you succeed. You can't control them, as we've seen, and even influencing them can be arduous. But if you can't avoid them, you'll have to deal with them somehow, something we'll discuss in greater detail in the next section of this book.

DISTRACTIONS AND TEMPTATIONS; IT WILL BE DIFFICULT TO DEFEAT THEM

And there's more to our environments than just the people inhabiting it. There are basically four different types of distractions; those you can control, those you cannot control, those which are annoying and those which are fun, but they all originate from our environment.

Some distractions are outside of your control, and they can be annoying (an office meeting) or fun (a dinner invitation). You can't prevent these, but you can be quick to return to work after either one with just a bit of self-discipline. Distractions which you can control can also be annoying (checking emails) or they can be fun (watching YouTube videos or posting on Twitter). Consider scheduling time for these distractions so they don't interfere with more important tasks. Set aside a few hours in the morning or evening for those distractions which you can control to make room for the distractions you can't control.

A study on distractions on focus included two groups; individuals who were promotion-focused and sought positive outcomes, and if individuals are prevention-focused, who tried to void negative outcomes. The study found that distractions, such as music, had little influence on the results. Rather, prevention-focused participants performed worse and enjoyed the task less than the promotion-focused test subjects.

But that doesn't mean distractions aren't still costly. You might spend one minute on your phone, but studies indicate that it may take over 23 minutes of wasted time to return to the task at hand.

Though distractions aren't always external. The left lateral prefrontal cortex of the brain may be impaired, making people more likely to succumb to the temptation of immediate satisfaction rather than long-term gain, which is just what a distraction often is.

LIVING WITH OVERTHINKERS AND PROCRASTINATORS

Often the problem of overthinking and procrastinating is part of the negative influence of others and your problem is having to deal with them. When you can't limit your exposure or try to redirect them in a positive direction, there are still good ways to deal with that negative influence, and to keep it from influencing you.

Don't minimalize their perspective. Overthinkers are obsessing, that's true, but telling them that doesn't help. One might be moved to try to reduce the scope of the problem to relieve the overthinking, saying basically, "It's no big deal." But procrastination and overthinking are as much emotional problems as anything else, as we've seen. So, trying to approach it logically won't work, and it may even make fixation worse as the one who overthinks takes offense. Then they'll overthink *that* too.

Similarly, don't reduce the potency of their feelings. Somebody who's overthinking something can't just get over it. They're emotionally locked in, and just like telling them they have nothing to worry about, telling them they have no right to their legitimate feelings will only make things worse.

A lot of anxiety is irrational, so there's no point in asking somebody why they're overthinking things. Again, it's not about reason, it's about emotion. Try talking to them about the emotions they're processing instead of the thoughts they're processing.

It also doesn't help to compare the overthinker's dilemma to anybody else's. These challenges are different for everybody and they don't all handle them in the same way. Nobody else's dilemma is going to be of very much use.

Strangely, overthinkers aren't often looking for solutions or recommendations, much as they would seem to be seeking that very thing. Because it's not about reason but emotion, overthinking and fixating on a thing is often a matter of emotional release. Sometimes, a person just wants to vent. They're more fixated on the problem than the solution. It may seem irrational, and it very often is. But overthinking and procrastination are emotion-based, after all.

In the same way, reassurance can be of little value to the overthinker. They're not thinking as much as they are feeling, remember that.

Overthinkers don't overthink everything, just some things. If you know a particular overthinker, reflect on the pattern of what they're talking about consistently. That will direct you in how to answer them.

Emotions tend to fester for the overthinker, which only makes sense. Very often, they're looking for a way to process all that emotion. But as a result of all that emotion and confusion, overthinkers are often exhausted, nervous, and agitated. Keep that in mind when dealing with them or avoiding them entirely.

But for now, let's take a closer look within to see what you can do to improve your own productivity and peace of mind.

3

STOP THE SELF-SABOTAGE! YOU, YOURSELF, ARE THE PROBLEM

S elf-sabotage, or the practice of either actively or passively preventing one's own success, can take a variety of forms. It can be active, such as substance abuse. It can be passive, such as with procrastination. But it's often dangerous and can be devastating.

Interestingly, the same things which motivate people to procrastinate also motivate self-sabotaging behavior in general; a lack of self-worth, a fear of success and failure, a desire for control.

Self-sabotaging is often indicated by the same red flags which indicate procrastination and overthinking; Prioritizing instant gratification over long-term benefits, avoiding necessary tasks, not prioritizing self, focusing on self-defeating thoughts.

And the same techniques you may use for procrastination and over-thinking are comparable to the techniques you'd use to deal with all the self-sabotaging behaviors; positive thinking, achievable goals to bolster self-efficacy, adjusting environment to limit distractions and negative influences.

YOUR HEAD IS FILLED WITH A LOT OF THOUGHTS, AND IT'S NOT HELPING YOU ONE BIT

Our days are filled with all manner of distractions and things which require our attention. This certainly doesn't do any good for those who tend to overthink or procrastinate. And all that clutter in our environment surely infiltrates our psyches. Remember that our environments mirror our psychological states.

But what kind of thoughts are streaming around in our brains, and how do we control them? The first step is to identify one type of thought from another and deal with each in the appropriate fashion.

There are basically three different kinds of thoughts: Necessary thoughts relate to your daily routine ("What am I going to have for dinner?" or "What's my website password?"), while waste thoughts - waste thoughts have no constructive use at all ("What if this happens?" "Why did that person say such a thing to me?") These are often related to past or future events, not events in the current moment, and concentrating on the past or the future instead of the present is a big part of both procrastination and overthinking.

Then there are negative thoughts, which are harmful to you and to others. Perhaps not surprisingly, negative thoughts are primarily centered on five common vices; anger, lust, greed, ego, and attachment.

The human brain exhibits signs of a negativity bias, the tendency to focus on negative thoughts. This was a survival tactic for our ancient ancestors, but in the modern era it's often a source of anxiety and depression.

Negative thoughts are generally inspired by unsatisfied expectations in disagreements, in laziness, racism, criticism, jealousy, hate, and an excess of power. They're born of bitterness, frustration, and dissatisfaction.

Positive thoughts, on the other hand, redirect our attention away from those common vices and toward the virtues of prioritizing love, peace, purity, joy, and power. These are the thoughts which drive our better selves and inspire our greatest accomplishments.

But of all the different kinds of thoughts, positive thoughts can be the most challenging to pursue, as they require a tolerance for discomfort, facing problems and low value tasks, and considerable self-discipline and inner peace. A person must be mindful of these challenges and reward themselves with praise for the small accomplishments, reassuring one's own psyche of self-efficacy and of the high value of sometimes-unpleasant tasks. It's a matter of will to a large extent, but that doesn't make it as miserable as it sounds. Remember to congratulate yourself for the little wins, remember how the little tasks add up to great accomplishments, that's not so hard.

Or consider thoughts as being in three classes. Insightful thoughts are used for problem solving, experiential thoughts focus on a task at hand, and incessant thoughts are the kind of chatter which distract us and cause us to overthink events in the past or the future.

Doctor Albert Ellis created an A-B-C approach to defeating incessant thinking. According to Dr. Martin Seligman, considered the father of positive psychology, a negative thought loop has three components; adversity, beliefs, and consequences. An unfavorable event creates adversity, which inspire narratives that become our beliefs. Those beliefs influence our actions, and those actions have natural consequences.

But you can add a fourth component, disputation, wherein you dispute the beliefs and correct them before they lead to their natural consequences. In other words, you can always talk yourself down from the pitch of your negative beliefs.

Your adversity, for example, might be in filing your taxes. There's a lot of miserable paperwork involved, even if you hire an accountant. You may tell yourself it's just too much to deal with, a narrative, and then believe that narrative. But you can dispute that belief at any time in the cycle simply by reassuring yourself that you can collect the documents and that your taxes will be filed on time. Believe it and do it and then *that* becomes the narrative.

Another way to disrupt incessant thinking is to replace it with a different type of thought; try experiential thinking instead, or insightful thinking.

Knowing what kind of thoughts you're having will help you to better control them and resist being controlled by them.

Bloom's taxonomy lists six types of thinking skills ranked simple to complex: Knowledge (remembering and recalling), comprehension (interpreting meaning and understanding), application (using old information in new situations), analysis (categorizing, differentiating, and examining), synthesis (combining different applications as necessary), and evaluation (critical analysis).

Negative thoughts can also be influenced by cultural (how a group expresses itself), genetic (how a family expresses itself), and physical considerations (how an individual express themselves). Racism may be an example of cultural negative thoughts, for example; a family feud may be a genetic negative thought, and a mental impairment such as bi-polar disorder may be creating negative thoughts born of a physical consideration.

But there are ways to counter these negative thoughts. Changing an external situation (such as divorcing an abusive spouse), shifting attention (to focus on the positive instead of the negative in a given situation) or re-appraising a situation (to see the benefit instead of the drawback of a certain event).

Researchers have found that genetics determine 50% of happiness, circumstances such as wealth and health accounts for 10%, Shifting or re-appraising, the internal and intentional efforts to achieve happiness, account for the other 40%.

There's also the cognitive triangle, which holds that our mental state relies upon the interworking of three major components of our psyche; feelings, thoughts, and behaviors. Each influences the other, and a sound footing for each is required for a balanced mental and physical state.

You may think you're hungry for a delicious but unhealthy cheese-burger because you deserve it, and that may encourage you to feel that you need it from sheer hunger, and your behavior is going to be to eat that cheeseburger. So, use a bit of mental discipline and replace the unhealthy cheeseburger with a yummy veggie-burger and let your feelings and thoughts continue as they are.

One great way to combat negative thoughts is to be aware of them and to employ *cognitive decentering*, which means you see a troubling event as just that, an event, and not a reflection of the self. Events are often independent of the self, as they happen externally and not internally. The key is to not internalize them and let them remain external.

DIAGNOSING YOURSELF: ARE YOU A PROCRASTINATOR? IF SO, WHICH TYPE?

As we have seen, procrastination is one of the classic methods of self-sabotage. But not all delays of performance are procrastination, only the chronic, habitual delaying of tasks. But we've also seen that there are different ways to procrastinate, different reasons for doing so, and so there are different ways of interrupting the procrastination cycle.

But let's take a closer look at different ways a person may procrastinate, and this comes down to personality types. Different people may form different procrastination personalities, if you will. For example:

Some procrastinators may be described as *perpetual lovers*. This people-pleaser may be stuck in a place of inaction for fear of hurting others or of being judged by them. We've already noted that fear of rejection is a big part of procrastination, after all. This person worries about how they're perceived, they seek not to be disruptive, they fear to be unloved or unwanted.

Some procrastinators are more like *error officers*. This is the perfectionist procrastinator who'd rather do nothing that do the wrong thing.

A *small player* protagonist is timid, afraid of the adverse effects of change, and procrastinating makes that possible. A *hidden gem* or *imposter* procrastinator may be insecure (such as a teenage girl or an incompetent worker or a liar) and a *poor thinker* procrastinator may be confused about social norms (a wealthy Christian perhaps). A procrastinator may also be a dreamer and not a doer.

Now that you know who you are and why you're procrastinating, let's move on to something everybody has, and nobody wants ... bad habits.

YOU'VE DEVELOPED BAD HABITS THAT YOU CAN'T GET RID OF?

Self-sabotage is basically a collection of bad habits; substance abuse, overthinking, procrastination, inaction. All comprise different sets of bad habits. If you overthink or procrastinate, the chances are good that you've developed some bad habits. And the fact that you're reading this book means that you want to get rid of them

So, let's get to it.

Some bad habits are very common to procrastinators of all types, so look out for these red flags.

Addictive habits like eating, drinking, or drug use has an immediate calming effect, but only contributes to procrastination. Procrastinators envy hard workers, and for good reason. They're also chronically unreliable, even for themselves.

Lack of physical fitness and weight gain are symptomatic of the procrastinator's lifestyle, as stress eating and no time to exercise prove a one-two punch to the body's chemistry.

You're always in a hurry because you're leaving things to the last minute, creating a constant rush to get them done. You only clean when you have an even more boring task to do. You may be easily stressed. You may stress clean only when a more stressful task needs to be done.

Too much social media is a big red flag.

Weekdays and weekends blur into each other, since you're spending your weekends finishing the tasks you postponed from the work week. But weekends are important for preventing burnout.

Oversleeping; it's a classic delaying tactic, even if you don't realize it ... because you're asleep.

How many times has your boss called you up for being late and you were sleeping? You know better.

You round up to the hour to forestall a task even for a few precious minutes. Instead of starting a task at 7:52, you'll wait until 8:00. At 8:05, you'll wait until 9:00.

You may be collecting smartphone apps, classic distraction devices.

You may be giving advice which you yourself don't follow. Why not? You've mastered through research that which you don't really know in practice. And that brings us to the Dunning-Kruger Effect.

Here's a helpful exercise: Make two lists; one of the numbers of your uncompleted plans and another list of episodes of your favorite TV show. If the first is longer, you know you're procrastinating.

Before we move onto the Dunning Kruger effect, let's talk about quitting bad habits. Habits easy to pick up but hard to quit are smoking and drinking. There are a number of reasons for this; some chemical and some psychological.

When you want to give up a habit, consider taking up the opposite habit. Instead of quitting smoking, take up the habit of becoming a nonsmoker. Replace that habit with another; walking, juggling, anything.

THE DUNNING-KRUGER EFFECT

Perhaps you've heard the old saying, "The more we learn, the less we know." It's about how humility comes with wisdom. Mathematician and Nobel laureate Bertrand Russell put it this way: "The fundamental cause of the trouble in the modern world today is that the stupid are cocksure while the intelligent are full of doubt."

So, researchers David Dunning and Justin Kruger set out to do an experiment on the certainty of one's own opinion and how it correlates to their actual ability. What they found was that certainty about a certain fact or circumstance was at its peak when the test subject was at the minimal level of competence. Increased competence created a lower level of certainty at first, but that rose with increased competence. The more we learn, the less we know.

The reason for this is a tendency to overestimate one's ability. Only education and wisdom can correct this overestimation. Many believe that those who are competent expect competence in others and therefore, estimate their own abilities as merely average. The less competent likewise expect others to be equally incompetent, and they can therefore assume that they are superior in their knowledge or capacity.

Furthermore, the study proved that the competent, when given an opportunity to self-assess, had no awareness of their incompetence. So not only do the incompetent overestimate their own abilities, they are impervious to any argument to the contrary. You cannot explain to an incompetent person their own incompetence. Largely it's a failing of logic. They cannot adequately use logic, as they are incompetent, therefore they cannot understand or accept it.

So, the first thing to do is make sure you yourself are not suffering from this widespread effect. Are you humble enough to know that you could be wrong, or that you might be acting from an emotional instead of rational place? How certain of your position are you? The more certain you are, the weaker ground you may be standing on.

And in dealing with others, if you can recognize the Dunning-Kruger effect, you'll know how to deal with those who are exhibiting it. Don't try to reason, as this person is not coming from a rational position. You may try to educate them, as increased knowledge is the only way to combat ignorant confidence, but don't expect them to digest your facts and be informed. They won't be moved by facts or logic because their position is not based on either one and their ability to see that is close to nil.

ARE YOU ARE OVERTHINKING IT? DO YOU KNOW WHY?

Overthinking comes in two forms; ruminating about the past and worrying about the future. Overthinking has its own set of bad habits too, so the better you recognize them the more quickly you can reverse them.

If you're an overthinker, you can't stop worrying or worry about things you can't control. You constantly reflect on your mistakes and relive unpleasant moments over and over in your mind.

Overthinkers tend to ask "what if..." questions endlessly and have difficulty sleeping because their brains won't stop circling around these negative thoughts.

You replay conversations in your head, regretting things you didn't say. You spend a lot of free time thinking about the hidden meaning behind things people say or events that occur.

You dwell on it when someone says something or behaves in a manner you don't like. You may also hold grudges and begin to feel paranoid that others are actively working against you. You spend so much time either dwelling on past events or worrying about the future that I often miss what's going on in the present.

Overthinkers are often overconfident in their own opinions and fixate on the opinions of others and are often pessimistic about what those thoughts are.

Overthinkers also fixate on what the deeper meaning behind some events might be, even when there might not be any deeper meaning or personal significance there. Overthinkers tend to want strict control over thoughts and actions and have little tolerance for spontaneity.

Some helpful ways to defeat overthinking can be used for other habitual patterns as well, including knowing and avoiding your triggers, be aware when you're doing it, and be aware of how essentially useless overthinking is. A forced distraction is another handy way to derail overthinking. Just apply your attention to something else ... anything else.

Since overthinking focuses either on the past or the future, focus instead on the present. Meditation can help, as we've already discussed.

A GOOD NIGHT'S SLEEP OR ONLY A FEW HOURS? EITHER WAY, IT WILL AFFECT YOUR DAY

Not getting enough sleep is a common form of self-sabotage and very common to procrastinators and overthinkers alike. It's often the result of spending long, last-minute hours completing unfinished tasks, or from tossing and turning while overthinking one event or another. But it's very detrimental to your mental and physical health and only furthers any downward spiral.

Most adults require between seven and nine hours per night, teenagers and children a bit more as they expend so much more energy during the day. While distractions like TV and video and the internet can rob us of our sleep, good diet and exercise can contribute to a healthy sleep cycle.

A healthy sleep cycle has been proven to have beneficial effects on metabolism, mental wellbeing, sex drive, and fertility.

On the other hand, sleep deprivation is known to make people vulnerable to reduced cognition, attention lapses, mood shifts, and delayed reactions. It is also connected to type 2 diabetes, obesity, heart disease, high blood pressure, stroke, overall poor mental health, and premature death. Sleep deprivation is also associated with impulsive behavior, anxiety, paranoia, depression, bipolar disorder, and suicide. Signs and symptoms include excessive sleepiness, frequent yawning, daytime fatigue, and irritability. Sleep deprivation may also weaken your immune system.

The digestive system is also vulnerable to damage from too little sleep.

Sleep affects the levels of the hormones ghrelin and leptin, which control the body's feelings of fullness and hunger. Leptin is an appetite suppressant and ghrelin is the body's natural appetite stimulant. Too little sleep reduces leptin and increases amounts of ghrelin. The result is midnight snacking, overeating, weight gain, and the resulting heath issues.

Sleep deprivation also reduces the amount of insulin, which helps to reduce blood sugar levels, released by your body after meals. It is also associated with decreased hormone production, such as testosterone.

The human body has an internal body clock which regulates the sleep cycle. The 24-hour cycle is called the *circadian rhythm.* The rhythm includes a sleep drive which gets stronger as the cycle works through. That sleep drive, called *homeostasis,* may have links to an organic compound produced in the brain called *adenosine.* Adenosine increases throughout the day and are broken down during sleep.

Light also plays a big part in the circadian rhythm. The brain's hypothalamus has a cluster of cells known as the *suprachiasmatic nucleus.* These cells process signals from the eyes to the brain during exposure to natural light. This is what tells the brain if it's day or night.

With the loss of natural light, the body releases the hormone melatonin, which induces sleep. Natural morning light stimulates the body to create the hormone cortisol, which we've already taken a look at. Cortisol promotes alertness and energy.

So, if your sleeping habits are irregular, consider the effect of light in the room, too much or too little. Improve your diet and exercise regimen and get at least eight hours sleep a night.

But there are a variety of tips and tricks to help ensure a good night's rest. You may consider establishing a realistic bedtime and do not vary. Go to bed at the same time every night, and at a reasonable time too. This will establish a healthy and consistent sleeping pattern.

Temperature and light have a big effect on sleeping patterns, so keep the lights low and the temperature reasonable. Some people disallow TVs, computers, and smartphones in their bedrooms to prevent distractions and unnatural light.

Since the body has to work to digest food and drink, a lot of experts recommend staying away from alcohol, caffeine, or large meals in the few hours before bed. Abstain from caffeine, alcohol, and large meals in the hours leading up to bedtime. Experts recommend avoiding tobacco at night, as nicotine is a stimulant.

Daytime exercise is good for expending extra energy and readying the body for a sound sleep. Taking a hot bath or meditating before bed can be good strategies for a better night's sleep.

Some people in our frenzied modern world don't have that luxury. Some may be shift workers, for example, and must wake and sleep contrary to the cycle of morning and night. These folks can still take measures, including naps, limiting shift changes, and maintaining healthy lighting.

The flipside of sleep deprivation is too much sleep, and that can be detrimental as well.

Hypersomnia is a medical disorder causing sufferers to sleep for extended periods at night and remain tired throughout the day. The condition causes people to suffer from extreme sleepiness throughout the day, which is not usually relieved by napping. Hypersomnia is associated with memory problems, low energy, and anxiety.

Depression, alcohol abuse, and some pharmaceuticals can lead to oversleeping as well.

Oversleeping can lead to a number of dangerous conditions.

Oversleeping can contribute to obesity. According to a recent study, people who slept nine hours or more per night were over 20% more likely to become obese over a period of six-years than test subjects who slept the standard seven or eight hours.

Oversleeping has a certain effect on neurotransmitters in the brain, including serotonin. This may cause people who are prone to headaches to suffer from them as a result of too much sleep.

Fifteen percent of people with depression sleep too much, and those irregular sleeping habits may only contribute to the problem.

One study showed that women who slept between 9 and 11 hours were almost 40% more prone to heart disease than women who slept the standard eight hours per night. Inflammation is also found to be more common in those who oversleep.

Diet can have a strong connection to oversleeping. If you oversleep, consider changing your diet to increase amounts of these important nutrients which you may be lacking: Theobromine, which is found in chocolate; dodecanoic acid, which is found in coconut and palm kernel oil; Choline, found in fish, shrimp, turkey, soy, eggs, and some leafy greens; selenium, common to fish, turkey, shrimp, beef, chicken, brazil nuts, and some whole grains; lycopene is found in watermelon, red cabbage, cooked tomatoes, red peppers, and guava; phosphorus can be found in eggs, sunflower seeds, lean meats, lentils, tofu, fish, and pumpkin and sunflower seeds.

Sleep is crucial to a healthy happy life, and either too little or too much can both cause life-threatening problems and be symptomatic of them as well. But sleep patterns can be improved in a few basic and easy-to-manage ways. And once you're more alert and well-rested, you'll be able to deal with the fears that are derailing your best efforts during your waking *and* sleeping hours.

4

THE FEAR INSIDE THAT YOU DON'T EVEN REALIZE THAT EXISTS

We've already taken a look at analysis paralysis, or what happens when a person is so beguiled by their choices that they make no choice at all. Largely, this is founded in the fear of making the wrong choice. Fear is at the heart of a lot of conditions like this one, and it's an emotion that's well worth understanding.

FAILURE, EVERYONE FEARS IT, BUT SHOULD YOU?

Nobody sets out to fail. But it happens, even despite our best efforts or intentions. George Washington and Abraham Lincoln faced failure after failure on their way to the crucial successes which ensured the survival of their country. Everybody faces failure in big ways and little; missing a job promotion, getting a bad report from the doctor, missing a green light or missing a deadline. So, failure is something we're essentially programed to accept.

What we really fear, however, is the shame associated with fear; the anger of others who may be disappointed, the resultant rejection which may occur as a result of that failure. It's the shame that gets us.

Unlike guilt, which makes us feel bad about our actions, or regret, which makes us feel bad about our efforts, shame is about who we are. It addresses the issue of self-efficacy which is at the heart of procrastination and overthinking. Our egos and self-esteem may feel threatened by shame in particular.

Overly critical adults often cause children to internalize these damaging mindsets. Fear-based rules and ultimatum cause many children to ask for reassurance and permission, and this need for validation often carries into adulthood.

Fear of failing can often inspire insecurities and uncertainties about what other people's impressions or interests are, what future possibilities may be or be limited to, makes you worry about what other people think about you. It addresses issues of self-confidence and encourages a general lowering of the bar in order to prevent the risk of trying and failing at something truly challenging and which would be thusly rewarding.

Failure tends to lead to overthinking as well, locking a person in a cycle of imagining a different outcome based on other things which could have been said or done. Fear of failure (or shame, as you like) can manifest itself in the physical, creating last-minute headaches, stomach aches, sweating, fever, and other things which may prevent action and thus the possibility of failure. Distractions and excuses for running out of time are two other classic symptoms of fear of failure.

One good way to deal with all this is to simply own it. Accept that failure and shame are the risk that anybody takes when they try to achieve something. Know the difference between failure and shame; accept the failure and reject the shame. There is an old adage my own father often shared with me: *"Always do your best. It's all that you can do, and all anybody can ask of you."* So, if you did your best and failed, what reason for shame should there be in failure? Failure is a steppingstone to success, after all. Another adage, popular among artists, goes: *"If you never fail, you're not really trying."* So, go ahead and fail and don't be ashamed. The real shame comes from not trying at all.

Oddly, it's often the most successful people who have a fear of failure, as their identity is so closely related to their success. For them, failure is the antithesis of life. It can boggle artists as well, creating mental blocks which prevent the very creativity they need to succeed.

While those mental blocks can be debilitating, others needn't be. There are things in life you cannot control, there are things which you can control. Focus on them. If your goal is to get a new job but you don't know the right people, focus on meeting the right people!

We've all heard of phobias, irrational and debilitating fears. Heights, snakes, enclosed spaces and wide-open spaces all their associated phobias. So too is there a phobia of failure; atychiphobia.

Atychiphobia is more than just a trepidation about failure or a concern about what others may think or even overthinking about what could be or could've been. It's a paralyzing fear which can overtake your body or mind. Physical symptoms of such phobias include quickened heart rate, difficulty breathing, tightness or pain in the chest, dizziness or lightheadedness, hot or cold flashing, digestive problems, trembling or shaking, or sweating. Emotional symptoms include intense anxiety or panic or anxiety, an overwhelming flight impulse, a loss of control and detachment from one's self, fear of powerlessness, or death.

Previous failures or a learned fear of failure can contribute to developing a case of atychiphobia. The phobia can also be a learned or inherited condition if passed on by a parent or friend in a process called *observational learning experience.* Even just reading or hearing about it may trigger informational learning and encourage manifestation of the phobia (or any phobia).

WE ALL KNOW ABOUT THE FEAR OF FAILURE, BUT DO YOU HAVE A FEAR OF SUCCESS?

It's almost a cliché, and one that's hard to digest. Who's afraid of being wealthy and successful? Well, it's like the fear of failure, which is more about shame. The fear of success is more about fear of change.

Introverts tend to have a fear of success, as they shy away from the extra attention success brings. Success can breed contempt and cost a person friendships. Success can be both fleeting and corrupting and is rarely all that it's cracked up to be. This is a kind of *backlash avoidance* which is behind a lot of cases of fear of success. It's about a fear of change and what that change might bring.

One may also fear that they don't deserve the success, and that they'll be revealed as an imposter and humiliated.

Signs of a fear of success include low goals, procrastination, perfectionism, quitting, self-destructive behavior, which should now be quite familiar to the reader. Ways to combat it should be just as familiar.

Explore the origins of the fear, the type of fear, the reasons for it. Own it and understand it. Exercising, dieting, having a sound sleep cycle, socializing, even journaling can help. Some recommend visualizing success, some using image boards to compile pictures of the things they wish to accumulate.

If you're having what is sometimes called a *panic attack*, there are ways to bring yourself back down to Earth. Take a walk, do some breathing exercises, call a friend for some support.

Journaling his highly recommended for the fear of success. It's recommended to take a half hour or so in the day, preferably at the same time every day, to write down whatever thoughts you may have on the fear of success; memories of the past, problems in the present, or plans for the future.

Fear of success, like all phobias, is an avoidance strategy. If you're afraid of rats, you'll avoid them. Avoiding praise or opportunities or even romances is how the fear of success may manifest itself.

The fear of success can actually take on familiar shapes, six different archetypes of the fear of success. Knowing which one mirrors your own feelings and understanding that archetype will help you overcome it and your fear of success.

- The *Goal Addict Type 1* is the overachiever. The goal addict is set on his or her goals high and proud of those achievements. For the Goal Addict type 1, failure is untenable but always likely.
- The *Goal Addict Type 2* is the other side of the goal addict coin; they set the bar low and succeed at that. For them, the risk of failure is fairly low.
- The *Disbeliever* is skeptical of success, that it can be achieved by him or her or by anyone else. For the Disbeliever, the risk of failure is almost nil, and any failure will be blamed on someone or something other than his or herself.
- The *Saboteur* is the counterpart to the Disbeliever. The Saboteur is, like the Disbeliever, a fatalist, but he goes into an essentially doomed effort with a positive, not a negative attitude. For the Saboteur, failure if virtually certain.
- *Half-Hearters* are somewhere between the Disbeliever and the Saboteur. The Half-Hearters will play along but contribute nothing, offer the unspoken skepticism of the Disbeliever and a counterfeit version of the Saboteur's willingness to participate.
- *Inventors* are centered on their own efforts but may resist being part of a bigger team effort. This sense of introversion works against their efforts to succeed.

NOTHING LESS THAN PERFECT KEEPS YOU POSTPONING YOUR DECISIONS AND ACTIONS

You hear it a lot these days: "Don't let the perfect be the enemy of the good." And it's as true for procrastination and overthinking as for anything else. Perfectionism is the enemy of the protagonist, for sure. We've already looked at how perfectionism works against the protagonist's best efforts to break the cycle and get things done in a timely fashion. What the perfectionist protagonist often forgets is that nothing is ever perfect, good is often good enough. What matters is that the task is accomplished to the best of the performer's ability, after all. That's always better than having the task not be completed at all.

How do you know if you're actually a perfectionist, and not just trying very hard? Perfectionists focus too much on the results and too little on the process. It doesn't matter how it gets done, as long as the results are up to par. Every achievement fades behind the next one. No victory is good enough, the work is never done. One project must follow the next, and none are ever really good enough. The perfectionist also beats himself or herself up over the results, any results; they're never good enough. The perfectionist is also a fast worker, not stopping until a job is done.

They sound like admirable traits, but they can cause a lot of procrastination and overthinking, among other destructive behaviors. The problem is that the procrastination is born of misguided activity, which is different than inactivity. The procrastinator may believe he or she is hard at work, but the task is not being accomplished for all the preparation being done instead.

And the higher the stakes, the greater the risk, the greater chance for failure and therefore, procrastination.

To combat the effects of perfectionism, one only has to reassure themselves that a thing doesn't have to be perfect, simply lower the par on the process and the results. Don't let the perfect be the enemy of the good.

Use design thinking to emphasize the process over the result. If the process is sound, after all, the result should be too. Give yourself time to be unproductive to rest your creative, physical, and mental resources.

Consider an action-anxiety rubric. In two columns, list a series of tasks, or actions, and the associated anxiety you may have with finishing those tasks. Pick the smallest one and resolve it. That will bolster your confidence and help break down the cycle of procrastination.

Stanford University psychologist Carol S. Dwick, Ph.D., believed that people generally had either one of two mindsets, fixed or growth. A fixed mindset focuses on current talents or skills or intelligence, believing that they are fixed in stone and cannot be developed. These people may believe, for example, that musical talent must be innate and cannot truly be learned. A growth mindset holds the opposite set of beliefs, that a set of skills or the breadth of intelligence can be expanded and improved. For this mindset, almost anybody may develop skills to become a musician or essentially anything else.

The fixed mindset tends to hinder growth and evolution, while the growth mindset has the opposite effect, encouraging growth and development.

We've looked at the basic causes of procrastination and overthinking and investigated the damaging effects and ways of coping. So, let's move onto Section 2 of this book and develop more specific solutions to break the cycle and eradicate the problems of procrastination and overthinking from your life forever!

II

DEVELOPING THE EXACT SOLUTIONS TO FIX THE PROBLEM

5

STOP YOUR PROCRASTINATING!

BE HONEST, HOW MUCH DID YOU PROCRASTINATE TODAY?

To be fair, you may not even realize you're procrastinating at all, never mind about how much. But a recent study indicates that only 18% of procrastination can be attributed to simple task aversion. So, what's going on with the other 82%?

Here we return to illusion of productivity. We may think we're busy, but we busy ourselves with tasks other than the one which needs to get finished. We're so busy preparing, we neglect to perform. But there are other, unconscious ways we procrastinate every day without even knowing it!

Blaming others is one way of procrastinating. Since so many of our daily tasks are reliant upon others also doing their part, it's altogether too easy for anyone to simply blame the performance of their counter-part. It is a passive/aggressive move, but very common with procrastinators.

We've already looked at how perfectionism can cause analysis paralysis, but this is also one of the unconscious ways of procrastinating. The perfectionist feels that they're moving slowly and surely, but often they're not moving forward at all. Worry, depression, fear of failure, and overthinking are common to the perfectionist protagonist.

Sometimes procrastination isn't related to the act at all, but the motivation; not the what but the why. Take marriage, for example. People have reasons (why) for getting married (what). They've committed to both, so they no longer question *why* they got married ... only *how* to stay married!

But procrastinators often can't answer the reason why, so they waffle. This could be why a lot of people put off the decision to get married. Under analysis, they can't answer the question of why they should do it, so they don't. This is increasingly common among millennials, among whom marriage rates have fallen drastically.

On the other hand, studies show that committed action produces more positive results.

As an exercise, imagine yourself in two months, and then imagine yourself in ten years. How will your choices affect you in two months or in ten years? Keep the long-term consequences in mind. Be aware of the subconscious ways you might be sabotaging yourself with procrastination and you'll be able to tackle them consciously.

One good way of dealing with unconscious procrastination is to keep a time log. For an entire month, write down everything you do and when you do it, in half-hour blocks if you can. At the end of the month, review the log and you'll see where and when you were less productive, even if you didn't realize it at the time. It will also illustrate why you were unproductive. You're bound to see patterns in time and activities.

When doing your time log, consider categorizing time spent for different functions. For example, you may spend your time doing paid work (your job), passion work (a side project), professional development (networking or job seeking), personal development (journaling or taking classes), relationships (friends, family, dating), play (shopping, surfing the internet or watching TV), wellness (exercise and self-care), support work (mentoring, volunteering), distractions (daydreaming) and maintenance (daily chores). Almost everything you do will fit into one of these categories. Your time log will help you identify how you're spending too much, or too little, of your time.

There'll be crossover, of course. Cooking may be classified as maintenance, but if you enjoy it, it can also be passion work, fun, or personal development. But when you're doing your time log, try to be as specific and as detailed as possible.

It shouldn't be surprising that time tracking apps are commonly available. *Hubstaff, HoursTracker, TrackingTime, Timely,* and *Hours* are just a few which offer different functions for tracking your time and the time of your staff, if you have one. Apps and websites which specialize in corporate time tracking for office management include

Paymo, Paydirt, Toggle, TimeTiger, Zoho, and others. Some of these apps are great for tracking budgetary and fiscal concerns as well.

Multitasking is one way we unconsciously procrastinate, for example. We think we're getting several things done, but none of them are being done as well as they could be, and studies prove that more mistakes are likely when focus is divided over several different tasks done at once. But that doesn't mean different tasks can't be done sequentially, one after the other. These are the tasks which get done successfully.

We've already seen how a strong support network can be an effective way to combat procrastination and overthinking. But a lot of people tend (unconsciously or not) to keep their professional and personal networks isolated. While there can be benefits to this, there are advantages to intermingling them as well. Friends can offer professional connections, and coworkers can become close friends.

OVERCOMING YOUR NEGATIVE SELF-TALK & PROCRASTINATION GOES HAND IN HAND

Negative self-talk, including self-blame and self-shame, self-deprecation, anything that breaks down your image of yourself. It's one of the great methods of self-sabotage and key to understanding procrastination and overthinking.

Negative self-talk leads to depression, lost opportunities, limited thinking, perfectionism, and relationship challenges.

By this time, you'll probably recognize what's become the procrastinator's motto: "I have to finish this long, important project. It should already be done by now and I need to plow through it."

But this is the kind of self-talk that can only fuel the procrastination cycle. But if you break this down, every part of the motto itself propagates the procrastination itself! The motto begins with *I have to*, but that's already shouldering the task with a lot of unpleasant associations. Nobody likes doing something they have to do. And there's an air of servitude to it, and nobody likes to feel like a servant. Instead, replace that with *I choose to*, which is far more empowering.

The motto goes on to use the word *finish*, but that only makes the task seem like one big thing. Instead, using the word *start* initiates a step-by-step process which can be more easily managed. In the same way, the long task should be reconsidered as a short task. If you're breaking the big job down into a series of smaller, more manageable tasks, then it *will* be a short task, right?

The motto's *important project* puts too much pressure on the performance and brings out the perfectionist protagonist in anyone. And since you've broken the big job down into smaller tasks, each one needn't be perfect for the whole to be a success. The *important project* becomes an *imperfect step.*

The motto goes on to say, *it should have been done by now*, and that may be true. But the verbiage is loaded with negativity. It implies failure and can only damage the worker's self-efficacy, a prime element of both procrastination and overthinking. Instead, replace that clause with *I'll feel terrific*. That's setting yourself a reward for accomplishment, an excellent motivator.

The motto closes with *I need to plow through it*. That establishes expectations of a long haul, which almost anybody would dread and then avoid. Instead, promise yourself, I'll have plenty of time for play. Again, you'll have something to look forward to, and you'll be looking ahead to long-term satisfaction instead of immediate gratification.

So, if the procrastinator's motto is, "I have to finish this long, important project. It should already be done by now and I need to plow through it," then let the non-procrastinator's motto be, "I choose to start this task with a small, imperfect step. I'll feel terrific and have plenty of time for play!"

Another kind of destructive self-talk is low self-compassion. The people that are hardest on themselves are less likely to be as productive as they could be. It's counterintuitive, because one might imagine that those who drive themselves harder would be more productive, but the resultant feelings of failure actually create the opposite effect. It creates stress and stress is harmful for the health and productivity of the worker, as we've seen.

Instead, practice self-compassion (few will offer you their compassion, after all). Forgive yourself for you mistakes or shortcomings, understand that you're doing your best and that nobody and nothing is perfect. But you have to do it deliberately. Self-compassion is the easiest thing to forget. You may have heard the old phrase, "We're hardest on ourselves." Well, make a conscious effort not to do that, and you'll be a lot happier, healthier, and more productive. Here's another old one: Guy goes to a doctor, bends his arms backward, and says, "Doc, it hurts when I do this." The doctor replies, "Then don't do that."

Of course, it's not always that easy. If you're plagued by negative self-talk, try asking yourself, "What am I feeling right now? Self-blame, self-shame? Am I indulging in negative self-talk?" If you are, don't do that. Instead, do the opposite and indulge in some positive self-talk. "Good job, buddy! Doin' great, sister!"

If that doesn't help, try something like, "May I be safe in this moment, may I be secure and accepted and loved." Don't forget to breathe in a deep, slow, steady rhythm. Then choose to do something which will bring you something pleasant and nurturing to put you back on track for more productivity later. But give yourself time to slow down and recalibrate.

To combat negative self-talk, learn to identify your inner critic and don't simply submit to it. Give it a nickname, like Debbie Downer or Mr. Grumpy Pants. Reduce its power over you and don't let the inner critic be constantly on your back. Stand up to them, cross-examine them, put their negativity to the test and you may just see it fall apart under scrutiny. He or she isn't real, after all. Thoughts aren't reality.

You can also set boundaries, even for yourself. Make it clear to your inner critic that some subjects are off-limits. You may also be conscious of negative language and replace it with neutral language. Replace "I hate ..." with "I don't like ..." Replace "I can't stand this ..." with "This is a big challenge." Negative language fosters negative thoughts. Words have meaning.

You may consider replacing your inner critic with an inner friend, one who naturally frames things in a positive fashion. Your inner critic may say, "You're worthless!" But your inner friend will say, "You're precious worthy!" Your inner critic may claim that you've fallen behind and failed in life, but your inner friend will reassure you that you still have so many accomplishments ahead of you.

You may reconsider your perspective. Will what's upsetting you now mean anything to anyone in five years? Does it affect anyone outside of your immediate circle? If not, maybe it's not such a big deal to generate all that negative self-talk.

And don't be afraid to say these things out loud. We've already seen how talking to somebody or even to yourself can be cathartic and helpful, and it works here as well. Give voice to it and that gives your new perspective even more power. Your ears will hear it, and that will help your brain to believe it.

It can be as easy as simply saying the word *stop!* When the negative self-talk begins, just tell yourself to stop, insist on it. Imagine a stop sign, or a door slamming shut to end the negative internal conversation.

Here's another interesting equation: *Events + Thoughts = Emotions*. An event strikes a person as troubling and they emotionally react. So, in essence, thoughts mediate emotions. You can't change the events, but if you want to control your emotional reactions, you need only change your thoughts.

But these thoughts don't occur in a vacuum. And there are general mistakes negative self-talkers make which only feeds the cycle of procrastination and overthinking.

Mindreading is the tendency to make assumptions about what others are thinking. These assumptions are almost always wrong, but they can be the subject of unending negative self-talk. Imagine being on a date and the other seems reserved. You may upset yourself with the certainty of a rejection, or it could be simple shyness.

Overgeneralizing is the tendency to assume that isolated events will repeat in a pattern. If the one date didn't go well, one may assume no date ever will. Fortune telling makes a similar error in perspective.

Magnification makes every unpleasant event a catastrophe. That date will be remembered as the worst date in history, and that will only propagate negative self-talk and limit future opportunities based on overgeneralizing.

Minimization is the other side of that coin, reducing every pleasant experience to coincidence or luck, but not due to personal achievement. Minimizing reduces the person as well as the event. The date may have gone well, but that could be attributed to a free meal, right?

Emotional reasoning allows a person to make decisions based on feelings instead of facts. Maybe the date went well, but this person just doesn't feel the right attraction or allows nervousness or fear of failure to prevent further engaging.

Black and white thinking leads us to exaggerate the nature of people and events to one extreme or the other. A bad date leads some to believe that dating itself is bad.

Black and white thinking often leads to personalization, when those extremes are applied to the self-talker, who takes too much responsibility for events outside of their control. The unfortunate dater may feel that he failed to charm his companion, when it could just as easily be something beyond their control. Some people just won't date others for a variety of reasons; race, height, other things nobody can control.

Labelling naturally results from all this negative self-talk. After the bad date, one may call themselves a loser. That's not a label anybody should have to wear.

Using the word *should* can be destructive too. It leads to overthinking about the past and the future, but that only stifles events in the present, as we've seen.

You can look for these mistakes in others' behavior as well as your own. You won't be able to control what others think and say, but you'll be able to avoid them and use other skills we've discussed in this book to better deal with them. Ask positive questions to counter the negative statements, for example.

And if you must be self-critical, do it intentionally and not habitually. It will give your self-critiques more validity and more effectiveness.

We talked about self-compassion, which is really a kind of positive self-talk. And just as there are drawbacks to negative self-talk, there are benefits to positive self-talk, including an increased life span, lower rates of distress and depression, better psychological and physical wellbeing, better cardiovascular health, improved coping skills and resistance to stress, even greater resistance to the common cold (still no cure though).

Positive thoughts flood your brain with endorphins, encouraging relaxation and contributing to alertness and a more centered psyche.

To encourage positive self-talk, consider identifying areas to improve, be conscious of your daily thoughts, embrace humor and a healthy lifestyle, surround yourself with positive people, and deliberately practice self-compassion and positive self-talk. It's easier than you think!

THE TRUTH ABOUT DOPAMINE, AND HOW TO 'HACK' YOUR BRAIN TO MAKE DOING 'HARD TASKS' SO MUCH EASIER (YOU MIGHT EVEN FIND YOURSELF STARTING TO ENJOY THEM)

Dopamine is a neurotransmitter produced in your body and used by the nervous system to transmit messages between nerve cells. Dopamine influences how we think and plan, strive and focus and find things interesting or pleasurable.

Studies show a connection between dopamine and several behavioral or biological functions, such as motivation, learning, heart rate, kidney and blood vessel function, sleep and mood and attention, lactation, and processing pain or nausea.

Too little dopamine has been related to schizophrenia, ADHD, and drug use and addiction.

Dopamine may be created by the body as a result of pleasure or even in anticipation of it, triggered by related sights and smells.

Symptoms of dopamine deficiency include difficulty concentrating, reduced motivation, concentration, enthusiasm, and alertness, poor coordination and challenged movement. Conditions associated with low dopamine levels include depression, Parkinson's disease, and dopamine transporter deficiency syndrome, or infantile parkinson-ism-dystonia, which causes uncontrolled movements similar to Parkinson's.

But too much dopamine isn't a good thing either. It can cause hallucinations, delusions, and mania and is associated with addiction, obesity, and schizophrenia.

If you're low on dopamine, there are a variety of ways to boost your levels.

Consider a change of diet to foods rich in tyrosine. These include meats, cheese, fish, soy, dairy, nuts, seeds, lentils, and beans. You can try a tyrosine supplement as well. You can increase magnesium levels by eating more nuts, soy, seeds, beans, and whole grains.

Avoid high-fat foods, sugar, caffeine, and processed foods. Correct harmful sleep habits and exercise daily. Use meditation, breathing exercises, and visualization to avoid stress.

You may even try natural nootropics like L-theanine and L-Tyrosine.

Neuroplasticity is the process of change in the brain in response to repeated experiences. So, if you use the techniques you've learned in this book, such as indulging in positive thought and adopting a healthier lifestyle, you actually train your brain to create more dopamine.

Exercise and productivity are good ways to burn through excess dopamine.

The section of the brain associated with automatic emotional reaction is the amygdala. This is where the fight or flight response occurs in times of great pressure. Often, to fight is to resist, and to take flight may take the form of merely ignoring a certain person or event.

Norepinephrine is produced, creating increased fear and anxiety, then adrenalin only makes the feelings worse. Dopamine, on the other hand, is the pleasure communicator. Experts have found that, to beat procrastination and overthinking, it's helpful to have more dopamine and less norepinephrine.

Our technique of turning one big task into series of smaller tasks will help us achieve that. A smaller, completed task encourages the brain to produce dopamine, and that dopamine fuels our further efforts. Conversely, the stress of completing one huge task forestalls the reward and thus the dopamine while encouraging the production of norepinephrine. Once again, it's a matter of changing your behavior before you change your thinking.

GET RID OF YOUR IMPULSIVE BEHAVIOR AND STOP DELAYING THINGS, THE SECRET TO GETTING AHEAD IS GETTING STARTED, AND YOU ALREADY KNOW IT DEEP DOWN (SO STOP DENYING IT!)

Impulsive behavior is generally not well planned, rather it occurs in the spur of the moment without thought to the consequences. Different impulsive adult behaviors include binging on food, liquor, or drugs; destruction of property, as in a temper tantrum; escalating problems and arguments, frequent outbursts; self-harm like cutting; physical violence such as punching; oversharing too much about personal or inappropriate subjects, and higher-risk sex.

In children, look for ignoring danger, interrupting, vocal aggression, physical aggression and grabbing.

Impulsiveness may be caused by personality or learned experience, or brain connectivity or function, but one cannot rule out the influence of genetics, childhood trauma, genetics, or physical changes in the body.

Mental disorders such as ADHD, antisocial personality, intermittent explosive disorder, borderline personality and bipolar may contribute to impulsiveness as well. Kleptomania (the desire to steal), pyromania (the desire to burn), and trichotillomania (the desire to pull out your own hair) are closely associated with impulsive behavior. Pathological gambling is one of the classic impulsive behaviors.

Brain injury and stroke may be contributing factors as well.

But there are times when impulsive behavior can be remedied. With an adult, consider walking through the possible scenarios of what may happen as a consequence. Take a moment to really think it through. The same is good for impulsive behavior in a child, though making a role-play game of it may make the lesson sink in a bit more effectively. They're children, after all.

As before, the environment is crucial, as it has a tremendous influence. In this case, seek out the triggers of your impulsive behavior and change your environment to exclude them as much as you can. Impulsive gamblers should stay out of casinos, for example. Impulse eaters shouldn't walk past the bakery. Change where you go, change your route to work to avoid the bakery, and you'll thwart those triggers and be able to change your behaviors.

As we've seen, the best way to get something done is to get it started. The journey of a thousand miles begins with a single step, as they say. And we've seen the value of breaking a big task down to small, manageable tasks. Well, the first of those tasks can only be one thing; getting started. The old saying, which has been attributed to a variety of sources including Mark Twain, goes like this: The key to getting ahead is getting started.

So, follow Nike's advice and just do it. It doesn't have to be great; it just has to be. You can correct it later if you need to, but at least you'll be engaged in the task and not stymied by analysis paralysis.

A lot of this will require self-control, and that can be improved. Like any big project, break it down into manageable tasks. Pay your credit card on time and enjoy the feeling of being responsible. The ensuing dopamine will propel you into the next self-control task, counting the calories of your next meal. You'll feel better and stronger and encouraged to move on to your next task of self-control, a trip to the gym. It's an upward spiral instead of a downward spiral, and one with all the positive mental and physical benefits to help you live a better life. You'll find that impulse control, procrastination, and overthinking are basically issues of self-control as well. And once you've conscientiously increased your self-control, you'll find tackling those problems easier as well.

APPLY DELAYED GRATIFICATION, AND MAKE TASKS URGENT USING ACTIVE PROCRASTINATION

A big part of defeating the cycle of procrastination and overthinking is delaying gratification. Immediate gratification is one of the leading factors in procrastination, as we've seen. But there are significant benefits to delaying gratification.

A Stanford University placed children in a room with a plate holding a single marshmallow. They were told they could eat the treat or wait 15 minutes and get two marshmallows. The ones who waited generally also did better on standardized tests, better behavior, and better health.

In your case, the delayed gratification which comes at the completion of a big task will be all the sweeter, and well worth waiting for if you break it down simply. Delayed gratification is at least twice as good as immediate gratification, but really, it's a hundred times greater, incalculably greater.

Think about previous experiences when you didn't wait and went for immediate gratification. How did that make you feel, what did you take away from that experience. Now reflect on a time you did wait or had to wait, like Christmas Day. How do you remember those experiences? Wasn't Christmas Day all the sweeter, more precious, for the wait?

The study also showed that children who were told to picture the marshmallows as little fluffy clouds had an easier time waiting, and those who were asked to describe the flavor and sensation of eating the marshmallows were less willing to wait. This suggests that emotion is a greater impulse trigger than reason.

Delayed gratification can also deliver the motivational factor that immediate gratification simply can't. Delayed gratification creates a goal, something to work toward. But immediate gratification cannot do this by its very nature, because it's immediate and goals are at least slightly longer-term in nature.

Buying a house, retirement, getting married, these are classic goals and all of them entail delayed gratification.

It's very likely that delayed gratification improves with time and maturity. An adult is more likely to value delayed gratification than a child. Baumeister's 2007 self-control and self-regulation theory (Baumeister, 2007), describes five different areas or domains of gratification delay. They include food, physical pleasure, social interaction, money, and achievement.

It's hard to resist a tasty snack, for example (food), a nice backrub (physical pleasure), a fun night out (social interaction), a quick bet (money), or a quick laugh (achievement). But these are the areas where delay is the most beneficial. Delaying food is healthier, delaying physical pleasure can lead to greater pleasure later. Avoiding a quick bet will save you the loss, a quick laugh may be inappropriate. Delay is only natural in these domains, they're a natural part of these things. We wait until mealtime to eat, until it's an appropriate time and place for physical pleasure. We make dates to go out and prepare for that event. We receive paychecks in two-week increments. We get promotions after years of work. We *have* to wait for these things.

Procrastination does have some positive aspects; however, active procrastination can be turned to anyone's advantage if they understand what it is and how it works.

Procrastination helps a person to learn how to manage delays, provides chances to reflect on your course and often results in making better choices. Procrastination may aid in prioritization and allow for smaller chores to get done. In its strange way, procrastination is the antithesis of impulsive behavior.

It took naturalist Charles Darwin 20 years to finish *On the Origin of Species*. Renaissance genius Leonardo da Vinci spent years fussing with his Mona Lisa. He was a perfectionist procrastinator.

Studies of college students indicate that many procrastinators are more competitive and ego-driven, whereas non-procrastinators are more task-driven.

Most people think of procrastination as being essentially passive; after all, procrastination is all about *not* doing a certain task, right?

But there is an active form of procrastination, when someone postpones a task deliberately and diverts attention to more important tasks. Those who actively procrastinate seem to prefer working under pressure. They are motivated by the challenge and often succeed in meeting deadlines.

Active procrastination has three major facets. The first is cognitive, when a person decides to procrastinate. The second is affective, when a person prefers time pressure. The third is behavioral, wherein they still complete the task on time.

Active procrastination is closely associated with multi-tasking. Active procrastinators tend to use task-oriented coping strategies in times of stress, avoiding emotional reactions. Passive procrastinators lean toward avoidance-coping strategies and rely on emotional reactions. Active procrastinators are driven by both intrinsic motivation, which comes from within, and the extrinsic motivation of a looming deadline. Active procrastinators often have a significant level of autonomy, self-reliance, and self-confidence.

But active procrastination must be learned, and here's a good exercise to help you adapt the more beneficial type of procrastination! Set yourself a simple task, let's say sending an email. Then put yourself in the place where that task is done, which in this case would be in front of a computer. Now don't do it, wait as long as you dare. Feel the emotions which result from waiting, accept that it will be uncomfortable, boring, frustrating, stressful. Let the feelings come ... and then let them go. You need to deal from a rational place, not an emotional place. Once the feelings have passed, begin the task. You've now mastered your emotions, and that's something the passive protagonist struggles with. Now you're ready to complete the task and get that email written!

As we discussed earlier, a habit is easy to give up and hard to quit. So often the best recourse is to take up the opposite habit. Instead of giving up meat, become a vegetarian. And the same is true for passive procrastination. It's habitual and a hard habit to break. But you can choose to be an active procrastinator instead, and let the good habit simply replace the bad.

POMODORO, THE PROCRASTINATORS' NEW BEST FRIEND

We've already discussed the notion of breaking down one big task into several smaller tasks, and the various benefits to this approach. But a more precise version of this approach is called the *Pomodoro Technique*.

The Pomodoro Technique recommends breaking big tasks down into 25-minute chunks, with a break of about 5- or 10-minutes. The technique refers to these 25-minute work periods as *Pomodoros*.

The frequent breaks keep you refreshed and focused, and the careful measurement of time keeps you focused and disciplined, while completing each Pomodoro gratifies and brings the reward of self-satisfaction and positive self-efficacy.

The Pomodoro is best implemented in stages; planning, tracking, recording, processing, visualization. Plan the day's events at the beginning of the day. Track your progress and new information throughout the day. Make a record at the end of the day to see the results of your progress. Also, at the end of the day, process that data into information by visualizing it so you can understand it clearly and use it to your benefit later.

To implement the Pomodoro Technique, use a timer to make sure you stick to the schedule. Start with a to-do list, in order of priority, and include a section for unexpected interruptions. Keep an activity inventor sheet too, to mark these things down, and a records sheet to list the data compiled throughout the day. And don't skip the breaks, they're important to keep you focused and vital throughout the day. Breaks are well known to have a lot of benefits. They let you take a step back and re-evaluate, rev up your brain, think of better ideas, and prevent exhaustion.

PROVEN STRATEGIES THAT WILL HELP YOU BEAT YOUR PROCRASTINATION

One advanced technique to control procrastination is Eisenhower's Urgent/Important Principle, which emphasizes using time effectively and not simply efficiently. This technique helps you to prioritize, to differentiate which tasks on your to-do list are important and which are more like distractions.

Being effective and not merely efficient means breaking down activities into two groups. Important activities relate to long-term goals, whereas urgent activities have to be dealt with immediately but may not relate to anything long-term. Knowing the difference will help you prioritize between the two.

Try it for yourself! Make a list of everything you do during the day, no matter how inconsequential it may be. Then break those activities into four categories; important *and* urgent, important *but not* urgent, *not* important *but* urgent, and not important *and also not* urgent.

When things are important and urgent, they may include things which are scheduled (important) and things which are unplanned (urgent). You'll want to schedule extra time to accommodate both. Important but not urgent tasks are vital for long-term success, so make plenty of time for these in your daily schedule. When something is not important but urgent, think about delegating the task if your time is taken up by something, anything, which is important. When something is not important and also not urgent, put that at the bottom of the list and reschedule until there is nothing in the first three categories.

Another helpful tip for beating procrastination is to break down your sense of time to the smallest increment. Instead of looking at your deadline as being three days away, think of it as being in 72 hours. It gives the delay a sense of being shorter and adds urgency to your motivation.

Think about how your work affects others. Very often, we lack self-care and self-support, but we're very caring and giving to others. Remember the phrase, "We're always hardest on ourselves"? Well, this gets to the root of that. So instead of thinking about yourself and your efficacy or insecurity, think about the others around you. If you procrastinate, how will that affect them, their careers and reputations?

You might also recast the deadline. If it's due on a Monday, give yourself a deadline of the previous Friday so you're sure to get it done even if you do procrastinate a bit.

Publicly committing to the deadline is a good way to put the pressure on. It's like giving your word. Your integrity and standing are great motivators! A motivational friend to check in and support you is also a potent strategy. You might think about making a gentlemen's bet with somebody that you'll finish the task!

Another good exercise is to pick a small task and give yourself five minutes to finish it. That'll be one small victory for you, one small defeat for procrastination. A lot of people have a favorite song which gets them excited for a particular task. Music creates emotional responses, and emotions have great power to inspire our behavior, as we have seen.

Now that we've made considerable progress defeating procrastination, let's do the same thing with overthinking!

6

OVERCOME YOUR OVERTHINKING!

DECLUTTERING YOUR MIND HELPS YOU RECHARGE YOUR BRAIN & RE-SHAPE YOUR BEHAVIORS & HABITS IN AS LITTLE AS DAYS

Previously, we looked at how the environment can influence thought and behavior. And in just the same way one's environment can become cluttered, so too can the mind. But decluttering the mind is a great way to overcome your overthinking.

So, consider your mental furniture; does it fit, do pieces clash? Are your mental appliances all in good working order, so you can cook when you need to and cool down when you need to? Does the décor really reflect who you are now or is there a lot of old stuff it's time to replace.

And while we're looking at the correlation to mind and environment, take a look at your actual environment. Is your house clean? Is your desk cluttered? Are you well-organized? These things will affect your psyche as much as they are affected by them.

Writing down your concerns is a great way to get them out of your mind, because those thoughts are now being stored elsewhere. Journal keeping has this benefit and lots of others, including giving you a chance to organize the things you're overthinking about and then solving or resolving them, turning negative thought into positive behavior.

Mental clutter is often caused by memories of things past; not pleasant memories, but grudges and unpleasant events which could perhaps have worked out differently. Let go of those things in the same way you'd throw out old magazines. They're not contemporary or relevant to your life in the present, and they take up a lot of space.

Multi-tasking tends to lead to a lot of mental clutter, because too many things are being tended to at once and they all can't be done to complete satisfaction. Multi-tasking clutters the worker's time and as a result, it clutters their mind.

Too much information is perhaps the leading culprit of mental clutter, and that makes sense. In our world today, we get more information and faster than ever before. The news cycles are shorter, the array of information is ever widening. So naturally we have too much information. But how do we resist that in this hyper-informative age? Limit your time on the internet or in front of the TV, be discerning about what you pay attention to.

Being decisive is a good way to combat overthinking too, because decisive action replaces the overthought which may create analysis paralysis. Being decisive also helps you prioritize, another key to breaking the overthinking and procrastinating cycles.

One great way to clear mental clutter is to meditate, that's a big part of what meditation is all about; clearing your mind and focusing. Deep breathing is a big part of meditation, and that practice on its own can be very helpful in ridding your mind of clutter.

As you might do with procrastinating, think about finding a supportive friend to talk to about your concerns. Speaking them will help get them off your chest and off your mind.

A healthy sleep cycle is important to sound mental health, and that's a key to breaking the overthinking cycle. Wake up early and go to bed at a reasonable time. Avoid things which will disrupt your sleeping patterns, as we've already discussed.

Getting in touch with nature is a great way to alleviate mental clutter. It's another case of the connection between environment and mental health. Once again, change your environment and you can change your whole way of thinking. The sounds of birds singing, a babbling brook, wind blowing through the trees, the smells and sights of the woods or even a public park, are refreshing and calming and should go far to helping rid you of that mental clutter.

A lot of people keep a mental inventory, which is a list of things one must do, things one should do, things one wishes to do. Once they're stored elsewhere, you can take them off your mental desktop, so to speak. Ask yourself how important each item truly is, to you or someone close to you. Keep revising that inventory as necessary, as old tasks are completed and new ones come up.

The brain is responsible for a variety of neurological and cognitive function, the latter group including language, attention, memory, visual-spatial skills, and executive function. But the brain can become bored with these functions and needs frequent stimulation. You can use specific challenges and relaxation acts to keep the brain functioning at its best.

Learning a new skill can be both a challenge and a relaxation act. Learning to cook, to paint, or play a musical instrument are great to both challenge and relax. Therapeutic yoga is also both challenging and relaxing, and very good for the body. Getting plenty of rest is a relaxation act (and often a challenge too) but it's vital to refresh the brain.

Problem-solving activities like puzzles and video games are a good way to keep the brain stimulated and eager to process new data. Expressing yourself artistically, as we mentioned earlier, is a great way to relax; dance, journaling, singing. It doesn't matter how good you're at these things either. This is not the time to be a perfectionist!

And don't forget to take time off for things you enjoy, as this balance is vital for an uncluttered and refreshed mind.

5 EASY STRATEGIES FOR OVERCOMING PERFECTIONISM & HOW THIS WILL REDUCE YOUR OVERTHINKING

Perfectionism, the drive to perform and produce flawlessly, may seem like a strong motivator, but we've already seen how it can actually impede productivity. It can also contribute to a lot of negative conditions, including depression, anxiety, obsessive-compulsive disorder, burnout, eating disorders, and suicide risk.

We've already seen that it's one of the major contributors to procrastinating and to overthinking as well. No conversation would ever have been perfect, no possible situation will ever be perfect. Nothing will ever be perfect, and if they are, that's probably owed to a dash of luck, something nobody can control.

As we did before, let's take a look at the language we use, because words have meaning and can drastically change our perspectives. For example, a perfectionist might say, "I didn't get an A on a test; I'm a complete failure." But an alternative might be something like, "Whatever the grade is, will it matter a year from now?" The perfectionist may say, "My haircut looks awful, I don't want to be seen." But the alternative may be something like, "People have bigger things to worry about, and it'll always grow back. With the way people wear their hair these days, probably nobody will even notice."

The attitudes are completely different, and so too will be the resultant behaviors.

But here are 5 concrete ways to help overcome your perfectionist overthinking:

- First, make a list of the advantages and disadvantages of trying to be perfect. You'll see right away how dangerous the disadvantages are (relationship problems, anxiety) and the advantages (better decisions after clearer reflection).
- Second, be more self-aware. If you tend toward perfectionism, substitute those thoughts with more humble thoughts. Focus on the positive in a project, not the inevitable little flaws.
- Third, as with procrastination, set a time schedule with limits and stick to it. It's a matter of self-control and self-care.
- Fourth, learn not to see criticism as a personal attack, don't respond to it defensively. Listen to the criticism and don't counter it, just digest it. If you've made a mistake, acknowledge it but don't beat yourself up for it. Everybody has the right to make a mistake now and then. Nobody's perfect, right?
- Fifth, set reasonable goals which you can accomplish. Setting huge goals which may be next to impossible is virtually setting yourself up for failure and disappointment, fueling the overthinking cycle.

A word about goal setting here. Perfectionists tend to set certain goals which only feed the perfectionist tendencies. Non-perfectionists set goals of a different sort. For instance, perfectionists often set goals based on what others expect. A healthier goal is based on personal wants or desires. Perfectionists believe their goal is perfection, while a healthier goal is based on relativity to the worker's abilities or recent achievements. The perfectionist may set a goal with the focus on the end result, while a healthier goal setting system may emphasize the pleasure to be found in the process; creativity and working with others, forming bonds, and so on. The perfectionist fears disapproval or failure as connected to the self, but a healthier goal setting mindset associates disapproval or failure with the project, not the workers.

And, when you're setting your goals, don't forget to be SMART. The goals should be specific, measurable, achievable, realistic, and timely; SMART.

Another good way to prevent perfectionism is to try to see a problem through somebody else's eyes. What would they make of it? What advice would you give to them? Remember, we're hardest on ourselves.

An exposure technique is when a person faces, or exposes themselves, to their greatest fear in order to conquer that fear. For the protagonists, those fears include rejection, failure, ridicule. So, a perfectionist can always deliberately achieve a little failure in order to discover how non-catastrophic such a thing could be. It may sound strange (unthinkable to some) but go ahead and mess up a little bit. Drop your train of thought during a presentation or wear a wrinkled shirt. Let an awkward pause go for a while longer than you might have. Then sit back and see what happens ... which will probably be nothing. Imperfections really only bother the perfectionist, and that's a vital lesson to learn to curb that often-destructive trait.

Another neat trick in dealing with perfectionism is to get a new hobby. You're not likely to master it right away, so you won't be expecting perfection ... hopefully. You'll be more drawn into the moment of learning and growing and not in the results or their consequences.

CULTIVATE YOUR MENTALITY TO ITS PEAK PERFORMANCE AND RELIEVE YOURSELF FROM ANXIETY AND NEGATIVE THOUGHTS

Perfectionists aren't the only ones who have anxiety and fear of failure, of course. We've already looked at some coping mechanisms for fear of failure and other problems common to procrastination and overthinking; be aware of the causes and triggers, reframe your beliefs around the goal to deemphasize the consequences, change your language and perspective from the negative to the positive, visualize potential outcomes, consider the worst-case scenario, and have a backup plan. Whatever happens, learn from it for the next time!

Ask yourself what you learned from a certain situation, how you can grow as a result of it, and find at least three positive things from the experience.

A SOUND MIND IS IN A SOUND BODY

We've talked about healthy and unhealthy diets and their effects on sound mental health, procrastination, and overthinking. The central organ of overthinking, the brain, has an even stronger connection to the body. The brain never stops working, not for one second during your life. So, it requires an incredible amount of energy, more than any other part of the body.

In fact, brain cells consume twice the energy of other cells. At between only two and three percent of the average person's body mass, the brain burns a full 20% of calories consumed.

So healthy diet and lifestyle are crucial for the brain, and for the cognitive functions the brain controls, as we've discussed. They provide the long-lasting mental agility needed to be productive. Ever have a big meal and then sort of crash? It's because overeating floods the brain with too much glucose. Too little glucose has a similar, debilitating effect.

Processed foods which are sugary, salty, or fatty take longer for the body to digest (a full three days for a McDonald's Big Mac). And that means less useful fuel for the brain ... and the rest of the body too.

For optimal mental and physical health, experts recommend avoiding anything processed, and eating your organic or natural foods slower to aid digestion. Your stomach takes about 15 minutes to send the message to your brain that you're full. Eating faster means you fill that gap with more food than you need, flooding your brain with glucose.

A few tips and tricks to eating healthier include substituting meats for vegetables in dishes like pizza or an omelet. Take coffee or tea without cream and sugar. Veggies and hummus can replace chips and dip at your next party. Cook at home, it tastes better and you know exactly what's in it and the circumstances under which it was made. If takeout is a lifestyle necessity, find the healthiest options. Taco Bell? Try

Subway. KFC? Well, anything's probably better than KFC unless you just eat the box. Even then ...

Running is an exercise and a recreational pastime which can have terrific advantages to a sound body and mind. It burns calories, builds circulatory and cardiovascular health, but studies show it offers brain support and enhances mood. It calms the mind as we concentrate on the basic movement instead of more complicated intellectual concerns. Running also uses up excess adrenaline or cortisol to diffuse stress.

Any exercise should be done in moderation, of course. Experts recommend 20-30 minutes at a time, two to three times a week.

Use a lot of the same techniques you used for procrastination (healthy sleep and diet, self-compassion, reflection, depersonalization) to help overcome your overthinking. And don't just think about it, do it!

7

SETTING GOALS THAT ACTUALLY INSPIRE YOU & ARE BUILT ON YOUR DEEPEST DESIRES

The great artist Pablo Picasso once said, "Our goals can only be reached through a vehicle of a plan, in which we must fervently believe, and upon which we must vigorously act. There is no other route to success."

So, have a goal which has a plan you believe in and act on. That really doesn't sound so hard, but there are facets of it which are easy to overlook. One of those is the goal. We've already discussed the use of short-term goals to achieve a single long-term goal by breaking up a project into a series of smaller tasks. But it's important to set the right goals, to be smart, or SMART (right?) about selecting our goals.

WHY SMART GOALS ARE NOT ENOUGH TO NUDGE YOU

You'll recall that SMART is an acronym for goals which are specific, measurable, achievable, results oriented, and time bound. But setting good goals alone won't do it. You'll need to put them into action. You'll have broken the project down into smaller units which can be achieved, sometimes called *milestones.*

To put this into play, start by making a list of tasks which will achieve each milestone. Use a timeline for this, as we've discussed.

We've already talked about apps for time management, but they have them for goal setting too! GTD Agenda (Getting Things Done) is one, and the basic $4.45-per-month plan allows you to track up to 30 goals and 50 tasks! *GoalsOnTrack, Profit, ClearCompany, 7Geese, Lattice, Sprigg,* and *Wrike* are others.

Because while smart (or SMART) goals are great, goal setting can be a lot more involved. Goals are not only crucial to the basic pattern of accomplishment, the first crucial step in that cycle, but studies have shown that they increase motivation and organization. And the more challenging and the more valuable the goal, the greater our efforts will be to achieve it and the greater the results of success will be.

Studies also show that clearly defined goals will lead to a superior performance. Research has produced a theory of goal setting based off five key principles: Commitment, clarity, challenge, complexity, feedback.

It really only makes perfect sense. The more committed we are to a task, the more likely we are to access and achieve. Commitment comes from proper motivation, such as long-term gain. Conversely, lack of commitment inspires lesser results, especially when the task is a challenging one.

Clarity is also key; the nature and purpose of the task, its value, its deadline. If a worker is confused as to what they're doing or why they're doing it, that greatly increases the chances of failure and inhibits the likelihood of achievement. But who could commit to something they can't even understand?

It's easy to see how these steps, like many in such equations, lead from one right into the other.

Once you have commitment and clarity, the goal should be challenging. It shouldn't be impossible, clearly, but boring and mundane tasks are the least appealing to the human psyche and most encouraging of negative mindsets which cause procrastination and overthinking. The human being likes to be challenged; it's how we built the pyramids and put a man on the Moon.

Complexity is important, as it must come in moderation. Challenge is great, but too much complexity interrupts the clarity we need to get the tasks done. But complexity does occur, often unforeseen and as a result of the accomplishing of the task itself, so make sure to budget a bit more time into a project timeline to account for complexity.

Feedback keeps the process and the progress moving forward during each of these stages.

A bit more on goals and how to set them:

Goal setting has been shown to improve academic performance up to 25%. Setting the right goal has been associated with optimal *flow state*, or *being in the zone*, as they say.

Research on college students found that optimism and hope made students better suited to setting goals and achieving their tasks. Students with high self-efficacy did better than those with less self-confidence. Either type of student seems more likely to be influenced by social forces in setting their goals.

So far, we've talked about goal setting as a more-or-less individual practice, but with bigger projects which require teams, a team approach to goal setting can be an invaluable approach! Research has proven this, but it only stands to reason. People inspire one another and come up with better ideas, and that encourages higher morale, clearer positive thinking, better results, in an upward spiral. This is often a worksite experience, face-to-face, but the same principle applies to virtual teams, who must do their collaborating over Zoom. But musical combos are playing together over such devices, theatrical productions are being staged all over the internet, even *Saturday Night Live* has done it. So can you!

Virtual groups should consider having a sort of director to centralize communications and keep things on track.

Before any goals are set, remember that the practice requires planning (knowing what the task requires for completion and how to break it down conceptually), self-motivation (we have to want to achieve the goals we're setting), time management skills (budgeting how long each smaller goal will take to achieve), flexibility (to adjust for complexity), self-regulation (to ensure effective performance throughout the entire task), commitment and focus (to know what you want and how to get it).

There are also different areas related to goal setting. Know which area you're treading, and you'll be better equipped to set the right goals.

Researchers identify two types of achievement goals; mastery achievement goals (focusing on skill development to achieve the goal) and performance achievement goals (focusing on ability of the individual). Basically, mastery is about the result, performance is about the performer.

Mastery goals tend to inspire workers to complete the task. Their focus is on the qualities of the task, not of the worker. They work hard to improve their skills, to master them, in the cause of the task, especially in times of failure. Performance goals tend to orient individuals to prove themselves. Results are often personalized and reflect on the qualities of the worker, not the results of the task.

Performance goals can inspire anxiety and reduce task performance, but mastery goals can increase involvement through ongoing improvement and self-evaluation. So, mastery goals can have a more positive influence on motivation and that influences goal achievement.

But not all research agrees. Results of one study show that mastery goals worked well for those with low achievement orientation, but performance goals reduced those subjects' interest in the task, leading to poor performances. On the other hand, high achievement-oriented subjects had positive reactions to their performance-focused goals.

Some research suggests that performance goals should be subdivided into two approaches; *independent* and *avoidance orientations*. When setting goals, individuals are driven either by a desire for success or a fear of failure.

As long as we're breaking up one big task (goal setting) into smaller ones, let's look at three helpful categories of goals. Time goals categorize into two smaller groups; short-term and long-term goals. Focus goals are the big ones, they're the ultimate long-term goals. Topic-based goals are generally things which happen alongside but as a part of the task. Paying your bills or filing your taxes may be one of these but would a long-term goal like buying a home.

A good exercise, as we've discussed but it's worth repeating, is to set a few short-term goals and then achieve them. That begins a healthy cycle of success to motivate you to move on to bigger tasks and likewise accomplish them.

Then build on that task. Do one task in a day, then set three for the week, ten for the month, and so on. Be realistic, but challenge yourself! It'll be worth it even if you don't do all ten in the month. You'll have done five or seven, and that's a lot. The old saying goes, *"I'd rather strive for a lot and achieve half, than strive for nothing and achieve it all."*

YOUR INSPIRATIONS AND DEEPEST DESIRES WILL GIVE THE REAL PUSH THAT YOU NEED

Desire is a powerful emotion and an even more powerful motivator. It's also a tremendous force for creativity. So, it only makes sense to plumb those desires to achieve our goals.

Desire and the energy it generates have a huge influence on our intentions and on our actions. But desire may be so close to fear that they become indistinguishable. Often when we think we're moving toward we want (desire), we are often moving away from something we don't want (fear).

Fear motivation focuses avoiding penalties for failure and can lead to feelings of compulsion or inhibition. Desire motivation is focused on rewards for success but can lead to low self-efficacy and feelings of helplessness.

So, know the difference between what is motivating your goal setting, and lean toward the desire and away from the fear.

GOAL SETTING STRATEGIES THAT WORK LIKE MAGIC

Making a plan is always a good way to encourage results. As we've seen, say it or write it down and it will tend to take on its own life, become its own motivating factor. Some researchers think of this as an *implementation intention,* and that makes some sense. It's your stated intention to imply your plan to achieve your goal.

But this is best broken down to specific, smaller tasks. Try this exercise and write this down on a piece of paper, filling in the blanks according to your specific desires or goals:

I will [BEHAVIOR] at [TIME] in [LOCATION].
  Some examples are:
I will sit in silence for five minutes at 6:30 a.m. in my
  bed before getting up.
I will study French for ten minutes at 8 p.m. in my
  bedroom.
I will go to the gym for one hour at 5 p.m. on
  Mondays, Wednesdays, and Fridays.

Once you fall into the habit of doing these things regularly, they won't seem like chores, but a natural part of your routine. Eventually, they'll be the kind of habits you won't be able to quit, and you won't want to.

But let's be honest, it all may not work out perfectly; as we've seen, it's rare that anything does. So, if you hit a stumbling block and can't make habitual one of your chosen planned activities, think about using the *if/then* approach.

Make a new list, stating the same goal which may not have worked out before. Then add an if/then function to the sentence:

If I sit in silence for five minutes at 6:30 a.m. in my bed
  before getting up, then I'll have a better day.
If I study French for ten minutes at 8 p.m. in my

bedroom, I'll have a better time on my trip when I
finally go.

If I go to the gym for one hour at 5 p.m. on Mondays,
Wednesdays, and Fridays, then I'll look great on
my trip to France.

Here's another run through of the if/then principle, also quite
practical:

If I don't sit in silence for five minutes at 6:30 a.m. in
my bed before getting up, then I'll do it at the
beginning of my lunch break, precisely at 12:00
noon.

If I don't study French for ten minutes at 8 p.m. in my
bedroom, I'll do it in the car on my ride to work.

If I don't go to the gym for one hour at 5 p.m. on
Mondays, Wednesdays, and Fridays, then I'll go
for two hours on Saturday and Sunday.

This approach allows for the complexity of things to intrude on your
carefully planned goals. Give yourself a backup plan and you'll be
much more likely to get the goal set and the task done.

The *if/then* approach can be directly applied to the overarching
problem of procrastination. To wit:

If I'm at my computer, then I'm working on the task.
Otherwise, I'm somewhere else.

If I want to procrastinate, then I'll remind myself how

good it will feel to get the task done and all the
good the accomplishment of the long-term goal
would do for me.

One overlooked aspect to goal setting which we should touch on here
is known as *calling a halt*. While we've been focused on setting our
goals and achieving them, it's important to recall one of the benefits of
overthinking, and that's a chance to re-evaluate. Sometimes a goal
which seems well-chosen proves out not to be the best choice. Sometimes a project is simply heading in the wrong direction. In that case,
the team may need to recalibrate. Goals may need to be reconsidered.
So, don't be afraid to call a halt to things, pull back and reconsider.

In setting a goal, you may consider creating a mantra. Anything
simple enough to repeat over and over and which will support your
mindset will work: *"I can do this, I can do this ..."* or "Everything's
okay, everything's okay ..." I personally combat a fear of driving over
bridges by singing a mangled version of a classic Pink Floyd song: "All
in all you're just another stretch of the road." Vocalizing gives power,
after all, and helps focus.

Here's another helpful acronym for setting goals and getting tasks
done! WAVE stands for Write, Act, Visualize, Evaluate. We've
already touched on all three, but acronyms are great ways to
remember things. Pretty SMART, right?

Don't forget that goal setting is something we all do in every part of
our lives; social, professional, creative, emotive. Setting goals can help
improve all of these, when used effectively and not just efficiently.

8

SKYROCKET YOUR PRODUCTIVITY LEVEL

FOCUS ON WHAT YOU'RE GOOD AT, AND BECOME BETTER ON IT

We've all heard of multi-tasking, the practice of doing several things at once. We've looked into it here and found it to be less than effective in most cases. Odd, though, that the original concept of single tasking now seems more like the novelty than the norm. Our lives have become so dense with information and tasks and a dearth of time almost force us to multi-task, creating failed tasks, less self-efficacy, depression, and so on.

Single tasking allows you to focus, to get into the zone for optimal performance. Multi-tasking clearly prevents that, as it's a result of sharp focus and nobody can focus as sharply on three things simultaneously as well as they can on one thing at a time.

So now we have to train ourselves to return to our simpler recent past and retrain ourselves to be single taskers. This may be a challenge, but it is well within your ability.

First, as we've said, start with small tasks you can reasonably accomplish. Then make sure you only do one of them, and don't even consider another until you've finished the first. Then proceed to the next task following the same rule. The key here is not to set aside a task, not to begin another or to tend to any external event.

Don't forget to break the task down into reasonable, smaller goals.

With your daily to-do list, do them separately and do the most important task first. This way, you'll have little to dread for the rest of the day. Do the next more difficult chore second, and the rest of the day will get easier and easier.

As with other techniques toward related conditions and corrections, work in blocks of time and schedule breaks. And keep an uncluttered desk for an uncluttered mind. This is particular important when retraining to be a single tasker, as distractions and complexities will rise up and challenge your focus on that single task.

Despite all the focus we've put on setting realistic goals and deadlines, when it comes to retraining to be a single tasker, it may be better to set *un*realistic deadlines. *Harvard Business Review's* Peter Bergman suggests that limiting time available for a single task at a third of what might be expected normally. The notion is that the time will exert pressure enough to force completion by keeping the worker more focused. This may make workers more productive and far less stressed-out.

If you're working on a project which requires a lot of research, use some kind of placeholder in all caps (*RESEARCH*, for example), and then do all the research in one clump at the end of the day. Alternating between writing and research may seem like two parts of the same task, but a lot of time is lost going in and out of the zone, recalibrating from one skill set to the other and back. And it's really just multi-tasking of another sort, if you really think about it.

Also, while doing legitimate internet research for your project, you may be tempted to succumb to the distractions of email, videos, and other things which inhibit productivity.

Be mindful of the fulfillment you enjoy by fulfilling a task. When that's a single task, the feeling comes sooner and can inspire you to more productivity. And when you're doing this single task, don't succumb to perfectionism. Let the task go when it's done and move on to the next … after a bit of a break, of course.

And once you've set about to become a single tasker, considering limiting that one task to do the thing you do best.

It makes sense on a lot of levels. We all want to spend our time doing what we enjoy, and those are almost always the things we're good at. All the great businessmen, innovators, artists, and athletes in history were doing what they did best, after all. And wouldn't the project, the company, all of society be better off if we all did what we loved?

It might be, but life's just not like that. We have to do things we don't like, things we're not particularly great at doing; that's a big reason why we procrastinate. So, a sound business model to fighting procrastinating and find the thing you're best at, master it, and apply that mastery. This is a personal journey each and every one of us must take on our own, and woe to those who don't take it at all.

You may want to volunteer at work or outside of work to give yourself time and space to indulge in your special skills. This will help develop them and also bring them to the attention of others, those who may allow you to use those skills at the center of your productive life. Volunteering is good for self-efficacy, high self-esteem, physical and mental health, a widening social circle, and it has a variety of other benefits too.

Don't be afraid to take a compliment. There's no shame in being good at something, and you may even learn about a hidden skill you didn't know you had. People generally don't see us the same way we see ourselves, and procrastinators and overthinkers are notoriously hard on themselves.

Scarcity Mindset is described as the fear of expunging one's resources and losing all. It manifests itself in a lack self-efficacy, when you may harbor self-limiting beliefs and negative self-talk. So, there's an impulse to hoard due to a lack of confidence in the ability to earn. It's a self-perpetuating phenomenon because it creates over-workers who earn less, and this only reinforces the scarcity mindset.

But you can always move past it just by recognizing it and changing your perspective. Stop imagining that the worst is certain to come, that failure is certain. Neither is true.

It's interesting (and a bit sad) to note that a lot people just haven't found what their given gift or gifts are, what they're truly best at. A lot of people go from endeavor to endeavor, school to school, career to career, never really finding their niche. If that's you, you'll want to take concrete steps to finding that special thing at which you excel.

Ask yourself, *"What skills have helped me thrive?"* Are you the type who always has a funny quip, is that your defense mechanism to avoid a variety of uncomfortable situations? Well, there's an old saying among comics: *"Funny is money."* You might be better suited to a position where writing is central. Are you a person who pushes forward no matter what, imbued with a determination that nobody stands in your way? You might be better suited to a career as a first responder than a librarian.

Ask yourself, *"What makes me feel strong?"* If it's bringing a smile to a child's face, a career in teaching may suit you better than a career in construction. If helping old people gives you that special feeling, then you'll know where to volunteer. If playing violin has always been your secret passion, go play it at the local retirement home.

You may ask yourself, *"What made me stand out as a child?"* So often, we lose touch with the things which were most special about our childhood. Were you an imaginative kid? Maybe that's where your true skills are.

Of course, there is often a big difference between what you're good at and what you're passionate about. It's great if those two things intertwine, but it's not always the case. My father was passionate about opera but could never write or sing in one. Lots of people are passionate sports fans but could never even think of playing professionally. Conversely, a person may have a certain skill at math, but not be passionate about their job as a mid-level accountant. Or you may have passion for something you're good at and then lose passion for it. This kind of burnout it common to teachers, social workers, and those in the mental health field. So be careful to know what you're good at, what you're passionate about, and which ones will truly help you to progress.

You may assume the answer is to choose what you're good at rather than what you're passionate about, but that's not always so (few things are). True, they say to lean to your strengths, and that makes sense. Do what you know. It makes good sense though it can also be a limiting mindset, keeping a person in the same, basically unsatisfying position for years. Doesn't sound like a very happy life, does it?

On the other hand, you can learn new skills in line with your passions, after all. Passionate about food but can't open a restaurant? Learn a little bit about writing or video directing and think about being a food critic. You may not know much about how to captain a powerboat, but if you long to live in a small yacht, you can learn those things.

Your secret skill could also be associated with your environment. Did you grow up with some special cultural influences which might impact your work for the better? Did you grow up hunting alligators in the swamps? You might write a book about applying the skills of the alligator hunter to those of the modern young corporate up-and-comer. Or you might lend your passion for nature to environmental causes, that's a win/win for everybody (and everything).

To this end, remember that it's better to be great at one thing than fair at several. Once you find the skill which will propel you forward, devote yourself to it and exclude distractions. Greatness comes from mastery, and mastery comes from a lifetime of diligence and hard work. Mastery is your long-term goal once you've found your special skill, not immediate gratification. Avoid the pitfalls of procrastination and overthinking when your special skill is involved; you can't afford to let that opportunity pass you by.

WHY SAYING NO TO PEOPLE AND CERTAIN PROJECTS CAN HELP YOU GET A LOT MORE DONE

Saying *no* isn't as easy as it seems. In fact, it can be quite difficult. In this people-pleasing world, nobody wants to offend anybody else. And since most people don't like hearing the word, they assume others don't as well, and they're generally right. *Yes,* is just so much easier.

But sometimes you need to say *no.* This whole book is about saying *no*, in fact; *no* to negative thinking and self-talk, *no* to being locked helplessly in analysis paralysis, *no* to unhealthy living. But those things weren't easy. And it only gets harder from there.

Saying *no* to others means risking rejection, isolation, ultimate failure. For the perfectionist protagonist, the word *no* hits them at the very core of their being, it's not merely a rejection of the project or task but an absolute rejection of everything they are, were, or ever hope to be. That's a shame, but not only does it not have to be that, but *no* can be a very positive thing. It sounds counter-intuitive, but it's true. Let's take a closer look at when and how to say *no!*

If you have to say to others, a basic rejection of an offer or suggestion, there are ways to make it more comfortable for everyone involved.

You might cushion it with kindness or a compliment. Always start with something good, such as, *"You've done a lot of work on this, and I admire that. Thank you."* Or you might try to find the one good thing you can start with. *"I like the way you've organized these tasks."* Then move on to your suggestion, correction, or rejection.

Then give your reasons for saying no, if you must. Explain it in a way which takes the focus off the other person. Instead of saying, *"You're just not right,"* consider saying, *"We're going to go a different way with it."*

Be brief during these exchanges, but there's no reason to rush or be brusque. There's time enough to make sure you've made your point with reason and kindness, but not so long that the subject is over-thought. Don't procrastinate the end of the meeting.

You might also think about replacing no with not now or not yet. That leaves the door open for further communications, better ideas to come across which you might find perfect for your next project. Remember, a *no* to the project does not have to be a *no* to the worker.

You may also offer an alternative. Instead of no, perhaps the notion has inspired you to improve the idea. If you can encourage the person to investigate other venues as yet undiscovered and then come back for another meeting. It tables the problem and makes way for a better answer. That's an example of using procrastination in a positive way, as we've discussed.

But if you have to say no, that can be a real trauma for some people. They can hardly bring themselves to do it. For them, or perhaps you, here are some tips and tricks to make it easier to do.

Be direct about it. No need to beat around the bush. Just say, *"No, I can't,"* or *"That's not for me."* And there's no reason to put it off either, that's procrastination of the worst sort and it will only increase your anxiety. Face the moment when it happens.

Remember that there's no reason to apologize or make excuses. Excessive people-pleasing should be avoided, lest you be overly reliant upon their approval. We've seen the trouble that can cause!

Don't lie, either. There's no need to, and it will only increase your guilt. Not only did you back out of something and disappoint someone, but you've also lied about it! Who needs all that anxiety?

If you don't say *no* now, you may be resentful of being embroiled in an unwanted task later. Don't let that kind of passive/aggressive behavior spoil your life.

However, there's no reason not be polite. You can always toss in a friendly, *"Thanks for asking though."*

You might want to practice saying *no*. Pretend somebody is asking you do something when you're alone, and say *no*. Try it with a friend. Break the big task down into smaller tasks.

Above all, keep in mind that your self-worth is not related to how much you may do for others, but for what you do for yourself.

What if somebody doesn't take no for an answer? Be courteous but assertive and simply repeat your position. Set boundaries and stick to them. *No* still means *no*, after all. Or you might turn it back onto the other person. If they insist, ask them why or explore other options with them.

Want to have your mind blown? If you can't say *no*, remember that every *no* is a *yes* to something else. Turning down a work project may mean saying *yes* to avoiding a disaster, or *yes* to more time with family and friends. So, you're not really saying no at all. It's not a matter of rejection, but selection.

HOW TO CREATE A SIMPLE TO-DO LIST THAT MAKES BEING PRODUCTIVE EASY, INSTEAD OF LEAVING YOU FEELING ANXIOUS

To-do lists are a powerful tool for organization, motivation, and tackling procrastination and overthinking, among so many other habitually negative behaviors. But an overreliance on them can be dangerous. Often times the lists themselves can become unmanageable.

Make sure every action on the list is important enough to warrant your attention. Get rid of the low-value tasks and more pleasant tasks for later if you need to. Start with a new list for every day and think about doing a weekly version too. This will keep the daily lists shorter and more well-organized.

There are three techniques to creating a workable to-do list.

You may start every day by picking one to three important tasks you'll focus on that day and make them your highest priority.

Or, at the end of the workday, you may select up to six tasks for the next day, in order of highest priority. Then put that list into action the next day, making sure they all get done.

Or you may choose 13 tasks of different priorities; one high-priority, three medium- and nine low-priority tasks. Complete them in order of high priority to low.

Instead of a to-do list, you might make a might-do list, to lesser the pressure and account for unexpected interruptions and distractions. Some recommend three columns per list; *to-do, doing,* and *done.* The approach helps the worker chart progress and rewards small achievements and reinforces self-efficacy.

Some people recommend publishing your to-do list, which we know can add motivation to get that list done. Others recommend drawing the list to embed it into your brain and excite your attention, though that may be time consuming. You can always put it on your to-do list though!

Other tips for better to-do lists include doing them in color to encode priority; red for important, blue for low-value, and so on. Or you may give each task a pleasant name; project flowers, project puppy dogs. It may take a lot of the misery out of the task, and it'll certainly will make it less intimidating. Words have meaning.

As it is with everything these days, there are apps and websites to assist with your to-do list management, including *Minimalist, Google Tasks, A Text File, Slack,* and others.

MULTITASKING MAY SEEM A WISE MOVE AT FIRST, BUT NOT ALWAYS. KEEPING A TIGHT LEASH ON HOW YOU SPEND YOUR ENERGY

While to-do lists have all kinds of benefits, some suggest they represent a misdirection of focus. A lot of professionals suggest that, instead of managing time, one should be managing energy. There's more than enough time, they suggest, but energy fails and that's the weak link in the chain.

You have 24 hours every day, after all, but you don't bring the same energy to every day. As we've discussed, your energy level is heavily influenced by your sleep and eating habits, lack of reasonable breaks and burnout, who we are with and what we think about, how we move or don't and how much or how little, our emotions, and our purpose or the lack of one.

Researchers believe that your purpose is the driving force of your energy. The greater your purpose, the more energy you will be able to muster for it.

It's also true that habits can either waste time and energy or increase both. Surfing the internet is a habit which may waste time and energy but taking a walk will not only increase energy for all kinds of biological reasons, but the time invested in it will increase productivity once work resumes.

In Spain, a three-hour siesta during the hottest hours of the day is a tradition, but that won't work in today's United States or almost anywhere else. There's too much to do. And sleeping three hours a day could have adverse influences on the individual in any number of ways.

But there are components of the siesta which could be quite beneficial. Quick naps during the day can be refreshing, after all, and revitalize the body and brain. Scheduled breaks, which we already know are beneficial, should be observed. But breaks should come in moderation, like all things. Too many breaks lessen productivity and encourage the protagonist /overthinking cycle of shame and depression and, ultimately, inactivity.

Remember also that energy comes in different types and can be wasted or harvested in different ways. Emotional energy is rooted in feeling beyond reason, mental energy is rooted in feeling which is within the boundaries of reason and intellect, and spiritual energy is rooted in the feeling in the strength of some transcendental belief. If you can recognize which type of energy makes you strongest, you can prioritize behaviors which foster that kind of energy. If emotional energy saps you, you can know to avoid the triggers for that kind of energy. If mental energy is your strength, foster it with reading and writing and learning new skills. If spiritual energy is what sees you through, spend more time volunteering at your favored place of prayer.

With all we've discussed, it shouldn't be a surprise that food has a tremendous influence on a person's energy. Processed foods, those which are sugary, fatty, or salty, don't nourish the system, they exhaust it with a labored digestive process. Organic foods and those rich is vitamins, nutrients, and natural proteins fuel the body with more energy. If you're governing your energy intake and outgo, diet is the first place you should go.

Caffeine is both a famous and infamous source of energy. A cup of green tea may contain up to 25mg of caffeine, the same amount of black tea up to 42mg, while a cup of brewed coffee may contain up to or more than 108mg.

Studies show that coffee offers a stronger rush earlier on, but that inspires a deeper crash later, while the lesser amounts of caffeine in tea offer less of an initial boost but a more sustained energy level.

Six ways of getting more from caffeine, and losing less to it, include drinking coffee or tea less, but over longer periods of time. Consider taking breaks between cups of coffee or tea for the same result. Drink water with your coffee to cut the caffeine rush. Stay away from those energy drinks, as they're packed with caffeine and are likely to produce an intense energy rush and then a deep, hard crash, probably sooner rather than later.

Eat well and don't drink caffeine on an empty stomach. That's a bit counter-intuitive because a lot of people drink coffee first think in the morning, before they have an appetite or a chance to eat any food. Still, this can lead to digestive problems and anxiety.

Now that we've learned more about setting goals, let's take a closer look at developing new routines!

9

LET'S DEVELOP YOUR NEW ROUTINES

WHAT YOU SHOULD KNOW ABOUT HABITS

Okay, we've looked at a number of aspects of procrastination and overthinking, and a few other things as well, mostly focused on reversing these established, negative behaviors. And, as we've seen, it's easier to pick up a new habit than drop an old one, so if you're trying to correct an old behavior, simply pick up the habit of the opposite behavior.

But bad habits like overthinking and procrastination, clearly our focus here, have to be well understood before they can be effectively manipulated. And to best understand a thing, you have to get to its roots.

All habits are often born of the three Rs; reminder (the trigger which touches off feelings that inspire the negative behavior), routine (which is the negative behavior itself), and reward (the emotion generated by the behavior). A big meal (trigger) may make you want a cigarette, so you smoke one (routine) and enjoy that rush of nicotine (reward).

It's pretty easy to see that you could break this cycle at any point in the cycle. Change your triggers and eat only light meals. Some people graze, or simply eat little snacks through the day and don't have any big, traditional meals. Some experts believe this is a healthier way to eat. Or you could change your routine by chewing a piece of gum instead of smoking a cigarette, which is a common substitute. This changes the reward from a nicotine rush to a slight sugar buzz, perhaps. It's still a reward, right?

Identifying triggers can be helpful. Take note of when the reminders, or triggers, strike by noting when the routines, or behaviors, occur. Do you smoke more at night than during the day? Take a closer look at why. Are you generally alone, or are other people involved? Is there one thing in particular which seems to inspire the desire to smoke? You'll find your triggers lurking in one of these questions. That'll help you root them out and either change or avoid them.

When changing your habits and developing new routines, keep in mind your inspiration for it, your long-term goal. That will give you motivation to carry on through the many smaller tasks which will be necessary to get the big task done.

And you can use the same techniques you've already started to develop! Enlist a friend for support and to be a sounding board, allowing you to vocalize your goals and give you advice you may need. Be mindful of what you're doing at all times, so you don't slip into old habits. Know what you're doing and why. Replace one habit with the opposite habit.

BREAKING BAD AND UNHEALTHY HABITS

What causes bad habits in the first place? Knowing the cause will help you discover the cure. As we often say, the answer is usually sitting right next to the question (or in this case, the solution is right next to the problem).

One aspect to the continuation of bad habits is the so-called *loophole*. Think of the loophole as the justification for the behavior. Being stressed out justifies the need for a calming cigarette break. Being bored often justifies overeating.

Now that you know what a loophole is, let's take a look at the different varieties of this insidious part of the bad-habit cycle.

First, there's the *false choice* loophole, where there's always something else to get done, It's a very common loophole. There's also the *moral licensing* loophole, where good behavior rationalizes the reward of bad behavior.

The *tomorrow loophole* is procrastination incarnate, putting off until tomorrow what could just as easily be done today. The *lack of control* loophole is the gambit of helplessness and submission to the bad behavior.

You may employ the *planning to fail* loophole, when you assume what you will try is doomed to failure and is unworthy of the effort.

The *This doesn't count* loophole provides convenient excuses like sickness or vacation to avoid the task.

The *one-coin* loophole assures us that there's always another chance, another day.

There's also the *questionable assumption* loophole, doubting the reason for the act; the *concern for others* loophole puts the blame on possible adverse reactions of or damage to others. The *fake self-actualization* loophole may convince you that there's no time to work toward long-term goals, that you must live only in the moment. This, of course, is a bastardization of the Buddhist notion of abandoning living in the past or future and to embrace the moment. The difference is in the grounding of the belief. For some, it's wisdom. For others, it's an excuse. If a Buddhist monk says this to you, give it some thought. If the person knows nothing of Buddhism or meditation and simply parrots the line, it's just an excuse.

There's also a biological aspect to bad habits.

The limbic system, the emotional parts of the human brain holds onto habits, as they are automated and easier to perform. But the prefrontal cortex controls the more disciplined activities. So, look to the limbic system as the root of your procrastination. Experts consider the limbic to be the older part of the brain and the prefrontal cortex the newer. Of course, all parts of a single brain are the same age. But emotional parts evolved first as a matter of evolutionary fact. Emotion secured survival and, slowly reason and discipline began to evolve based on the emotional core that was already there. Think about the discovery of fire, the domestication of animals, the change of prehistoric lifestyle from monadism to establishing fixed communities, or clans. We were emotional first, and we still do tend to put emotions first because that part of the brain has been developing over a longer period of time.

Stress and boredom are the root of a lot of bad habits. We're looking for an amusement to counter the difficult or tedious parts of our lives, and those are crucial in the procrastination and overthinking cycle. So, while it's difficult to avoid these triggers, or reminders, you can always change your routine. If distractions are a common respite from boredom, take a walk instead. It has every benefit of health and mind which watching YouTube videos of dancing cats simply doesn't. Conversely, we've already seen the detriment of spending too much time in one place. If you're not working, why use your workstation for amusements? Change your environment, a practice you should recognize by now as being amazingly impactful on any frame of mind.

Another well-used technique is to visualize. Imagine yourself not having to rush out for cigarettes first thing in the morning. Visualize yourself warm inside with your family and friends while others stand out in the cold smoking their cigarettes in isolation.

And don't personalize it. You're not your habits; you can always improve.

And there are a few concrete steps and exercises which will help you break just about any bad or unhealthy habit.

You might consider leaving yourself Post-it notes to remind you to curb a certain routine. If your long-term goal is to go to Paris, but you want to lose 20 pounds first, just write *Paris* on a Post-it and stick it on the refrigerator door.

Just as we used *if/then* to moderate and modify our goals, try *but* here. You may smoke, *but* you're going to quit smoking. Don't just accept that being a smoker is part of who you are, like your height or your skin color.

We've seen the value of time tracking, and that's of value here too. When you feel the reminder, or trigger, or when you indulge in the routine, or behavior, write it town. Be detailed, not vague. Note the exact time, place, who you're with, what is happening. Then examine your log and note the patterns. The triggers will rise to the surface by appearing more commonly on your log.

THE POWER OF HEALTHY HABITS WILL HELP YOU CONQUER YOUR OVERTHINKING AND PROCRASTINATION

We've talked about replacing one habit with its opposite. And what are the opposite of bad habits? Good habits, of course, healthy habits instead of unhealthy habits. Some of those unhealthy habits include drinking too little water, eating too late at night, getting too little exercise and/or sleep. Eating too much sodium is another unhealthy habit, as is eating processed foods. A lot of times, so-called *fat-free* foods are worse than natural foods with natural fats.

Eating lunch at your desk and using too much olive oil are common unhealthy habits. Skipping dessert is also less healthy than it sounds, and keeping an unclean kitchen has lots of hidden health risks.

And these are all easy to correct. Keep your counters clean, have a piece of cake, stay away from any food that comes in a colorful box or plastic wrapper. Don't eat after eight pm. If you can do those few things, you can counter a number of common unhealthy habits.

You may not have heard of the *two-minute rule*, but it tells us that any new habit should only take about two minutes to do. This approach basically breaks down any task to its first, simplest step. Reading at night becomes reading a single page. Thirty minutes of yoga becomes simply pulling out the yoga mat. The habit of studying for class becomes simply opening the books and leaving them open. Running three miles becomes a walk around the block.

It's another way of breaking down the big task into smaller, manageable tasks with concrete goals, the rewards of which propel further performance. Naturally, this is a stepping-stone technique! Stopping at two minutes of anything won't get you far.

This micro-habit technique is popular with a lot of experts, who also assert that there are habits that most successful people share. These are the healthy habits you can adopt to counter the negative ones.

Practice passion do what you love even if you don't do it professionally and do it passionately. Read and workout to keep your mind and body strong and clean. Save money. Have a mentor and be a mentor. Be mindful of relationships and of selfcare. Work even when you're not inspired and quiet the so-called monkey brain, that part which is so easily distracted. Do this by using a mantra. Donate time and money to inspire the feeling of self-efficacy. We've touched on all of these in this book, so it's remarkable to note that the world's great corporate successes employ them. And you can too!

Here's another helpful way to break old, negative habits and picking up new, healthy habits that will stick. First, make the old habit invisible, remove all cues. Then make it unattractive, remind yourself of all the negative aspects. Make it difficult, physically inconvenient. Make it unsatisfying, visualize the negative results and the immediate unpleasant consequences.

To make good habits stick, do basically the opposite. Make the healthy habit obvious instead of invisible. Make it attractive by visualizing the benefits of the healthy habit. Make it easy instead of difficult, make in convenient. Then make it satisfying by visualizing all the benefits and positive results and the immediate pleasurable rewards.

Apply cigarette smoking versus gum chewing and see how easily it works! Go ahead, I'll wait.

See? And it works every time, as do most of these techniques.

DAILY MEDITATION & MINDFULNESS CAN REVOLUTIONIZE YOUR MOMENT-BY-MOMENT HAPPINESS

Daily meditation and mindfulness are powerful techniques for creating healthy habits and they're both very healthy habits on their own. Meditation may help you better understand your mental and physical pain, help you connect better to yourself and others, lower stress and improve focus, and reduce negative self-talk and the easily distracted monkey brain.

Health benefits associated with meditation include lowered blood pressure and improved blood circulation, a lower heart rate and slower respiratory rate, reduced anxiety, stress, and perspiration, lower blood cortisol levels, a heightened sense of well-being and deeper relaxation.

Meditation has great calming effects. Research has shown that EEG activity actually decreases during meditation. Meditation also helps you to recharge so you have more energy throughout the day.

Meditation increases blood flow in the brain and may have positive neurological effects. It can also reduce the need for sleep. Meditation may slow the aging of the brain and enhance muscle control, emotions, and the senses of seeing, hearing, and the ability of speech.

Meditation helps achieve flow, or being *in the zone*. That, in turn, helps get more done and defeats procrastination. Medication has been proven to increase students' test scores up to eleven percent.

There are volumes on the shelves of our local bookstore about it, or on Amazon, but let's take a look at these practices as they relate to bad habits, goal setting, procrastination, and especially overthinking.

There is a variety of different meditation styles, each with its own benefits.

But first, how do you learn to meditate? In mindfulness meditation, we're learning how to pay attention to the breath as it goes in and out and notice when the mind wanders from this task. *Returning to the breath* strengthens your ability to be mindful and to pay attention and remain focused.

Meditation may provide space in your mind and in your life, and that's what the overthinker needs most. All you need to start is a comfortable place to sit, some patience, and some self-compassion (sometimes the hardest part).

But be prepared! Meditating may make you sleepy, and it may be hard to find the time. It's well worth it though!

Paying attention to your breath teaches you to return to and remain in the present moment, abandoning the past and the future. That's what the overthinker needs most.

In mindful meditation, you pay attention to each breath and concentrate on only that. In and out, the natural connection of inside and outside. Keep focusing on it as you do it, don't let your mind wander. Fix on the simple, natural, nurturing act of breathing.

How do you learn to meditate? In mindfulness meditation, we're learning how to pay attention to the breath as it goes in and out, and notice when the mind wanders from this task. This practice of returning to the breath builds the muscles of attention and mindfulness.

It's that simple, but it does require practice. The more you do it, the better you'll be and the better the results will be.

To practice this powerful technique, first sit down and get comfortable. Prepare yourself to be sitting still for the next few minutes. Set a time limit, especially when you start. Like all things, break the big task down into manageable smaller tasks.

Now focus on your breath. Where is it going inside you? Are you filling your lungs or just your nose? Is your breathing regular? Do this for about two minutes, then inhale and exhale deeply and slowly.

Repeat this cycle for as long as you can, and you'll note the amazing benefits. You can vary the cycle too, using a fixed focal point to focus on instead of breathing.

Mindfulness is a word we've been using a lot, and it deserves a closer look. Mindfulness is that consciousness of behavior which we so often overlook. Bathing, eating, driving, social interaction, even work, become collections of automated behavior that we just don't think about. Breathing is one of these; it's automatic, you don't have to concentrate on it in order to make it happen.

But a lack of mindfulness creates sloppy work, bad health habits, careless or reckless driving, failed relationships, because we just don't think about what we're doing. We're repeating the same things we've done for years, and in pretty much the same way.

Ways to be mindful are easy to apply! Practice mindfulness during routine activities like sweeping or cooking. Practice mindfulness first thing in the morning for a mindful start to the day. But don't restrict your mind from wandering, that's part of the exercise. You'll become skilled at bringing yourself back into the focus of mindfulness.

But keep it short. You don't want to stretch yourself too thin with this exercise and be mindful of every little thing. One thing a day to start.

Practice mindfulness while you wait; long lines and traffic are great times to refocus. You may want to pick a place or time, such as your coffee break, to practice mindfulness.

So, it takes a deliberate decision to be mindful of these things, of all things if you can be. Meditation uses mindfulness to guide focus. Mindfulness of something as basic and automatic as breathing is the perfect way to sharpen the skill of being mindful, strengthening the mindfulness muscle, which we can then use to greater effect in other aspects of our lives.

Body scan meditation is a simple and powerful technique too, which can be combined with any mindful meditation regiment. Just sit down where you are comfortable and sit quietly. Instead of focusing on your breath, or a single focal point, you'll be focusing on your body. Start with your feet and just feel them (not with your hands). Feel the blood running through them, the bones and tendons and muscles. Now scan upward through your legs, surveying their condition, feeling them as a part of your body. Progress upward through every part of your body to the top of your head It's a way of reconnecting with yourself, of becoming more comfortable in your own skin.

Walking meditation is another way to strengthen mindfulness. You don't have to be sitting down. You may focus on counting your steps, up to 10 then back again. The important thing is to fix on something simple, to clear your mind and not clutter it. And given all the health and mental benefits of walking, this is a beneficial technique in several ways. Do watch where you're walking, however!

Loving-kindness meditation has its own challenges for perfectionist protagonists and negative self-talkers as it relies on self-compassion, hard for some to achieve. Loving-kindness meditation focuses on the positivity of the person meditating, on their lives. It celebrates good-heartedness and open-mindedness and forgiveness.

Try using a mantra to practice loving kindness, such as, *"May I live in safety"*, *"May I have peace, joy,"* *"May I live with ease,"* *"May I have physical happiness* (or health, or freedom from pain, depending on your needs)."

Spiritual meditation allows you to focus, not on your body or your breath or on a fixed focal point, but on God or whatever is the source of the mediator's spiritual faith. The goal is to be closer to oneself by being closer to god. Potent oils and incenses are often used, such as frankincense and myrrh, sage and cedar, sandalwood and palo santo.

Focused meditation focuses on other things; counting beads, a song. Mantra meditation uses a simple monotone to focus on, like the famous, *"Oooouummmmmmmm ..."*

Transcendental meditation is perhaps the most well-known. It builds on mantra meditation but includes more sophisticated mantras specific to the reader.

In Visualization meditation the meditator imagines themselves at that place where the goal is achieved, visualize what that will look like, focus on that.

You may have questions about meditation. If you do, you're certainly not alone! Here are a few commonly asked questions about meditation and, of course, their answers.

Q) What if I have an itch?
A) Resist it if you can, try to scratch it with your mind. Failing that, scratch it. You're trying to focus on other things, and an itch is a terrible distraction and one that's easy to deal with.

Q) Should my breath be slow or fast or regular?
A) Just relax and breathe. A natural breathing rate will find itself, most likely. Breathe too fast and you may pass out!

Q) Should I close my eyes?
A) If you like, but it won't make using a focal point much easier! It could make walking therapy absolutely hazardous. A lot of people do close their eyes during mindful meditation, yes. If you do, take it easy. There's no reason to clamp them shut. Make it easy.

Q) Maybe I just can't do this?
A) Everybody thinks that, and it doesn't stop them. It shouldn't stop you. You *can* do this, but it will take practice. Remember that nothing worth doing is ever easy.

Q) Should I meditate alone or in a group?
A) Either, depending on your preference. Consider both!

Q) Is there an optimal time of day to meditate?

A) Not really, as long as it remains convenient, but tomorrow doesn't count!

Q) What should I do if I become aroused?

A) Accept that your mind will wander and just bring yourself back to your point of focus. No worries.

Q) Should I involve my pet?

A) As long as you don't interact with your pet, it's fine for them to sit quietly with you.

Q) How long should I meditate for?

A) It's more about regularity than duration. As long as you do it every day, it can be for as little as five minutes. Make it convenient and attractive.

Q) What should I wear?

A) Something comfortable.

DON'T BECOME A SLAVE TO TECHNOLOGY, YOU SHOULD BE THE MASTER OF IT

Truly, information is at the heart of the technological age. But some information is useful, some merely entertaining. Generally, the more entertaining a certain piece of information is, the less useful it's likely to be.

Either way, technology is everywhere in our modern world, and it is one of the most potent sources of distraction and brain clutter there could ever be, fostering monkey brain and triggering all manner of behaviors. But we do need our phones and computers and the internet just to survive. Banking, remote working, connecting with family and friends, technology is at the heart of our lives and that's not likely to change anytime soon.

There are lots of benefits to reducing your tech time. Studies show that computer light can be harmful to the eyes, posture can be adversely affected. Staring at your phone prevents you from fully interacting with others, leading to missed opportunities. Time spent playing app games on a smartphone could be better spent daydreaming or meditating or conjuring up new goals to set and tasks to achieve. It encourages rudeness when a person meets with another and then spends the whole time on the phone with somebody else. That's always been considered discourteous even in the time of land-lines. And the internet is rife with all kinds of misinformation and dangerous people who could easily victimize the unwary internet surfer.

So how can you prevent yourself from becoming a slave to all this tech?

With streaming sites like Netflix, so-called *binge watching* has become a trend. But that doesn't mean you have to sit in front of the TV or computer. Clean, cook, sew, do laundry, work out; there are all manner of useful chores can get done while the Trailer Park Boys are up to their goofy hijinks.

If you feel yourself overwhelmed by too much information, go back to our established tips and tricks. Write down everything you watch and categorize it, ranking it by quality on a scale of one to ten. Then eliminate the bottom 20%. Or, if that's too drastic, pick three things of the bottom 20% and temporarily replace them with something else. You can always switch back.

Say no to three things this week, it almost doesn't matter what they are. As long as you're eliminating these tech-oriented distractions for this week and see how you feel about it next week. Include all this in your log or make a new one just for this experiment.

Some people are visual learners, some learn better from hearing things. Know which you are and emphasize these things in your tech time. Visual learners may prefer to read a book, audio-oriented learners might spend more time with an audiobook.

Cut back on the quantity of all your tech time. Log up your time on phone, computer, iPod, and tablet, and reduce all by 10%. It's an uncomplicated way to reduce your use of, and dependence on, high tech. You can spend that time meditating, walking, visiting with friends, or enjoying a healthy, nourishing meal.

Some researchers, individuals, and families have adopted a new protocol for dealing with the intrusiveness of high tech on their lives, the new etiquette of the digital era:

No phones during mealtimes, social gatherings, or driving. No high tech for kids under a certain age. No phones as music players; use an mp3 or other dedicated music player. No high tech in the bedroom, or strict time limits. No ring-tone notifications. Those are for phone calls. No smart watches unless it is for health-oriented purposes. No phone app notifications. Keep two computers, one for work and one for play. Keep the play computer out of sight until appropriate.

Now that we've got a better grip on managing our energy and our tech, let's take a closer look not just at managing time, but using it wisely ... hopefully without too much high tech!

TIME MANAGEMENT IS THE ANSWER TO MOST OF YOUR PROBLEMS

Time management is at the heart of what procrastinators and over-thinkers suffer from and seek to overcome. While it's true that energy is important to manage on its own, time management remains essential. And the tips and tricks to help become a better time manager are the same as the others. It's amazing how this relatively simple set of skills can be applied to so many levels of the same challenges, and to different challenges altogether.

Time management has amazing benefits. You'll get better results, faster. You'll be more productive. You'll waste less time and avoid complications and conflicts. Better time management helps clear your slate for leisure time, which is good for a balanced life. That makes you calmer and gives you more opportunities to avoid stress. In the workplace, you won't miss deadlines or be late for appointments, your focus will be more fixed, you'll avoid stress. You'll avoid penalties for failure and enjoy greater rewards for your success.

Time management encourages patience, focus, organizational skills, decision-making, plan-making, motivation, goal setting and self-awareness.

So, as we approach other challenges, we look at time management as something which can be handled in (hopefully) recognizable steps. It begins with effective planning and is followed by setting the right goals and objectives. Reasonable deadlines and delegation of responsibilities (in a team setting) before prioritizing tasks in order of importance and then allocating the proper amount of time to that activity.

In general, use what you've learned to be a better time manager. Make lists and time logs, prioritize tasks, set the right goals and so on. Be selective and abandon perfectionism. Focus on the task, not yourself.

But what if you're a shift worker or have some other job which makes time management even more difficult? Let's take a look.

You may not have heard of the 80/20 rule. It holds that 20% of our efforts wind up resulting in 80% of our outcomes.

LEARN TO PRIORITIZE WHAT YOU'LL DO NEXT

Prioritizing is a big part of getting things done, as we've already seen. So, let's take a closer look at how to best prioritize our tasks. You may recall the matrix we used about priority, that there are urgent tasks and important tasks. Important tasks are more closely associated with long-term goals, and urgent tasks are more short-term. Some are important but not urgent, some urgent but not important. Use the matrix help prioritize your tasks, as we've seen. It's just another example of how these principles operate across the board. Master them, and you can apply them to every level of everything in your life.

We've been talking about breaking things down into smaller parts, and (hopefully) it's worked. But there's another way to look at it, especially if you're prioritizing. You might want to gather your smaller to-do lists into one big master task list. This will help you see them all in a single context and you'll be able to prioritize each list. That's what prioritization is all about, right?

There's a funny turn of phrase, *eat the frog*. Attributed to Mark Twain, who said something like, "If your job is to eat a frog, it's best to do it first thing in the morning." It's a beautiful illustration of prioritization. Get the biggest, most unpleasant job done first, it'll make everything else seem easy as pie ... which is a lot tastier than frog!

Some people prioritize by alphabetic notation. The so-called *ABCDE method* rates tasks in that order of priority. It may work for you.

Now let's move into the third section of this book and continue to look outward, rather than inward. Our next subject, your support partner!

III

IMPLEMENTATION

10

FINDING AN ACCOUNTABILITY PARTNER COULD SUPERCHARGE YOUR SUCCESS

WHY AN ACCOUNTABILITY PARTNER CAN MAKE THE CHANGE THAT YOU ARE HOPING TO HAVE IN YOUR LIFE

We've already looked at the many benefits of having a support partner. They can provide advice and compassion, a sounding board and a commitment board. They can impart good advice, help you reason out bad ideas, set goals, change self-efficacy. A support or accountability partner is invaluable.

Think of all the successful institutional pairings in history; any US president and his vice-president, any golfer and his caddie, any boxer and his coach, any superhero and his sidekick. Scuba divers go down using the buddy system. Most incredible of all, people are still getting married! The buddy partner works, but ... why?

They curb procrastination and urge a mentee to stay on track. Once that behavior is learned, it inevitably takes hold. Support partners keep you motivated and help ensure you meet your goals. They offer a different, more enlightened perspective, and can positively influence goal-setting and other crucial steps. And, as accountability partners, they hold you accountable if you falter and to stick to your deadlines. A lot of people need that support, and they should have it ... and they can get it!

THE CHOOSING PHASE, THE QUALITIES OF AN ACCOUNTABILITY PARTNER THAT YOU SHOULD SEEK

How do you best find or choose an accountability partner? It may not be as easy as it seems. Some in your line of work may be too competitive, or fear giving up their secrets. Others may be too busy or just too selfish. Some aren't cut out to be mentors either.

First of all, make sure you choose your accountability partner based on your goals. If you want to succeed in advertising, look for somebody who knows the field. A Catholic priest may not be the best choice. If you're putting a corporate team together, you might seek out a high school football coach, or somebody skilled in team-building who might bring a new and competitive voice to your efforts.

Once you know what you're looking to do and who might be best to help, ask your friends if they know anybody who might be interested in helping. Coaches love to coach; teachers love to teach. Consider a professor at your local university who specializes in the field you're pursuing.

Joining classes is a great way to find an accountability partner. The gym is a good way too or volunteering at any number of places eager for some extra help. There you'll find people ready and willing to share their time and influence, just like you are. If you were working at a food bank and some young person asked for your support, you'd give it, right? Right.

And these days, you can find the support you need online. Whatever you're doing or whatever subjects your project may touch upon, there's a Facebook group or an online forum about it. That is an invaluable resource for finding not just one support group but dozens, and from all around the world! There's never been a better time to be supported by people in this way. Beware of trolls, of course.

There are even apps like *Fitstream* to help build support and accountability groups.

One part of the process of choosing an accountability partner, of course, is being one. Having a mentor and mentoring someone else is still key to our regiment, up and down the board. Each has its distinct benefits.

And for the stage in life when you want to mentor, consider what it takes to be a good support partner.

You'll have to be supportive. Sure, you'll start off with that impulse, it's at the heart of what you're doing. Still, you're not there to be a contrarian, to play the devil's advocate. Support means support.

You'll want to focus on the goal, not the person. Always depersonalize these things.

You'll want to prioritize listening and understanding. Don't just nod and smile but invest yourself in these challenges and draw upon your experience to be a truly valuable resource. That's why you're doing it, after all.

You'll want to keep the lines of communications open in both directions. And when you communicate, be thoughtful in your counsel. Your mentee will be listening and just may follow our advice, so be careful what you say and how you say it. They may personalize your advice, especially if it's critical of the work.

Once you commit to a mentorship, don't quit. They may quit you, but if you abandon the mentee that could trigger feelings of failure, of anger, and could begin the procrastination or overthinking cycles which we're all here to suppress.

And be open to sharing your life. That's where your greatest wisdom is, after all. And it will help build trust and make you a better mentor.

11

HOW TO TACKLE THE BIGGEST & MOST IMPORTANT PROJECTS THAT WE ALL LOVE TO PROCRASTINATE ON

CHANGE COMES WITHIN AND YOU MUST CHOOSE IT YOURSELF

Elizabeth Kubler-Ross created the change curve looking at how people dealt with a terminal diagnosis. It measures confidence and morale against looking to the past and looking to the future. The four stages of the curve are information, support, direction, and encouragement. Interestingly, they correlate to the five stages of grief: Denial, anger, bargaining, depression, acceptance.

It sounds a bit complicated, but it works something like this: In stage one of the curve, information. When the diagnosis comes, the patient is apt to suffer a loss of a high degree of confidence and experience denial. The second stage lends support to the patient, though confidence and morale are likely to plummet and anger more likely to rise. The third stage of the curve, direction, tends to raise the patient's confidence and morale as they explore new options. Stage four of the curve, encouragement, tends to boost both morale and acceptance.

The model can be helpful, not only with a terminal diagnosis, but any change. Divorce, news of pregnancy, the end of a romance, a job loss or even a job promotion! When change comes to you, think about these stages and understand what stage you're in and how you're reacting to it emotionally. Understanding these things will help you to control them, in fact it's the only way to control them. Knowledge is power!

There's an old saying which was made very popular in Alcoholics Anonymous, and it's known as the *serenity prayer*:

God, grant me the serenity to accept the things I cannot change, the courage to change the things I can, and the wisdom to know the difference.

And it's effective for all kinds of change when that change is hard to deal with. But let's look at this time-worn bit of wisdom a bit more closely to see how we can apply it to our personal and professional lives.

When you're managing personal change, it is vital to accept the things you cannot change. Think of the overthinker, who constantly replays bygone disagreements, saying in their minds what they didn't say at the time, wondering what might have been said to create a different outcome. But that cannot be changed. The past has passed. So, it's a waste of time and creates all manner of negative behaviors. In looking ahead to manage your own personal change, keep this part of the serenity prayer in mind too. You'll never be taller; you'll never regrow that hair. Don't even waste your time trying. Instead, focus your time on the next part of the prayer.

If there are things you *can* change, then make a plan to change them. If a degree would increase your chances of success, make a plan to earn one. That big task would include just about every technique we've discussed in this book, but that would be a thing you could change. First, you'd need a plan. Losing weight, quitting smoking, getting control of your temper; all of these can be changed, but they need a plan which includes small goals leading to the ultimate goal, a timetable, and other analytical steps as we've already discussed.

Knowing the difference is what stops the overthinker, as the things which can't be changed are often perceived as if they could be. Future events can be affected by what we do in the present, right? Some of them can be, yes. Then again … you control your finances, but not the overall economy. As too many people learned, you can do everything right in preparing for your future, but economic forces may undo your years of diligence. You can control how much you spend or save, but you can't control a recession.

But you can be a strategic thinker and prepare for contingencies. We talked earlier about including time for complexities which arise suddenly, and when you're managing your own change and your own future, give yourself a margin for the unexpected, and then be prepared to accept it when it happens.

Abraham H. Maslow, famous for his *hierarchy of needs*, once said, "One can choose to go back toward safety or forward toward growth.

Growth must be chosen again and again; fear must be overcome again and again."

It's clear how this applies to managing your own change. Personal growth and change don't just happen, and if they do, they become twisted and unruly. You (or anyone) must take control of that growth and change, shape it properly, manage it constantly. Also, personal growth is not a one-and-done deal, it's a process. So be prepared to embark on a long journey. If you're not prepared, you're likely to backslide. It happens to a lot of people who mistake the first step for the entire journey.

Or you may think of personal growth as a savings account which only grows as you contribute to it over time.

Personal growth, in fact one could say that the person you are, is defined by the choices made. Better choices make for more personal growth which makes a better person. And, as almost always, there is a cyclical nature to this construct. The lesser choices make for less or no personal growth which makes a lesser person who makes even lesser choices which make for even less or no personal growth which make an even lesser person who makes further lesser choices and so on. The cycle feeds itself and the spiral either goes up or down. Which direction it goes is up to you.

So, when you're making these choices which will drive your personal growth up or down, you may ask yourself, *"Am I going to regret this choice? Is this in line with my integrity and my values? What will I gain from this and what will I lose?"*

You'll know what the answers are. It's just that most people don't ask the questions before they act or react. It's always wise to step back and consider before any action is taken. That's a technique we learned from active procrastination, which is actually a positive behavior.

SHOULD YOU RELY ON YOUR IMPLICIT MEMORY, YES OR NO?

Implicit memory can be described as engrained, automated into your behavior. One of its subsets is procedural memory. Tying your shoes or riding a bike are capabilities stored in your procedural memory. Implicit memory is a higher grade of this kind of memory, often called unconscious or automatic memory. Athletes, dancers, and musicians know it as *muscle memory*. Years of repetition make certain functions, like throwing a football or playing a musical chord, virtually automatic. Recalling words to a song is another example or driving a car.

There is also explicit memory, wherein a conscious effort is made to retrieve memories. Thoughts of historical facts, events on a vacation, people you knew all reside in your explicit memory. Unlike implicit memories, explicit memories are vulnerable to loss.

And there are two types of explicit memories. There are memories of specific events, like your wedding day or what you did last week; these are episodic memories. Semantic memories include names, dates, historical facts, general knowledge which is not so particular to episodes in your life. Episodic and semantic memories, the two subsets of explicit memory.

Research shows that stress and mood have a strong influence on the formation of both semantic and episodic memories, and so does age. It's pretty well-known that both types of explicit memories fade with time and the effects of aging on the brain. But it's also true that semantic memories may become unreliable as well. They're still more reliable than explicit memories, but our faith in them as being just about 100% may not be as accurate as we thought.

But there are ways to test implicit memory. Researchers have three ways to measure the loss of this essential function.

In the word stem completion test, the subject is given several alphabetic letters and instructed to provide a word which starts which each of those letters. Seems fairly easy, right? Try it now: A, C, E, O. I'll wait. Okay, while you did yours, I came up with *apple, chalk, example, owl.*

In the word fragment test, the subject is presented with an incomplete word and asked to complete it, such as *restaura__, bycic__, free_ay, au_omob_le,* and so on. If you squint your eyes, you can see the complete word based on your implicit memory of those words.

There's also the anagram solving test, where the subject is given a jumble and instructed to rearrange them in the proper order: *takecj (jacket), repnosltaiy, (personality).* That last one would make a good game show!

There are also different types of implicit memory.

Procedural memory, which we've already touched on, includes learned behaviors which become automatic, tying your shoes or riding a bike.

But there's also *priming*, wherein reactions become automatic. How many people were afraid to go into the water after JAWS? That was because the movie primed them to be fearful of sharks. There's also classical conditioning, which trains the subject to automatically respond to a certain stimulus, like Pavlov's dog. If you don't know, Pavlov rang a bell and gave his dog a treat. He did it repeatedly, so that the dog was conditioned to anticipate the treat when the bell rang. Then he rang the bell and didn't give the dog a treat, and the dog waited patiently for the treat.

Implicit memory is a kind of long-term memory, and long-term memories have a big impact on your activities and behaviors. They're formative.

Short-term memories, on the other hand, last for less than a minute. They may become long-term memories with some effort (the name of someone you just met) unless they're absolutely spectacular (a first kiss).

ESTABLISH YOUR SELF-DISCIPLINE AND SELF-CONTROL, AND DON'T LET ANYTHING HINDER YOU FROM WHAT YOU MUST DO

Finding motivation is a crucial step in establishing and developing your self-discipline. You may be motivated by life's necessities, such as feeding yourself or your family or obtaining safe or better shelter. You may want to help others, once you've seen to your own hierarchy of needs. You may want to achieve something that will transcend you and speak to others whom you will never know. You may simply want to have a happier life, to enjoy yourself more.

Here are a few questions to guide your decisions to apply reason to your desire and increase your self-discipline. Make a list (naturally) of what things you want and how many. Are they reasonable things? Are the amounts reasonable? Maybe you can cut the amount in half. Would that rob your life of its joy? Would your head explode?

Ask yourself again how much you want the object. Would you commit a crime to get it? What would you sacrifice to have that thing? How much do you want the object? How much joy do you get, or will you get from the object? Is it worth the inherent risk? How much will it hurt not to have it?

Answering these questions will help you establish and improve your self-discipline and that will help with everything else you do. Don't wait for it be resultant of your other efforts, make it the wellspring of the other campaigns. They'll work together, but self-discipline really is a good place to start.

Are you lacking in self-discipline? Do you have overwhelming desires to do something you know is bad for you? Do you succumb to those desires? How often? Are you disgusted at the idea of doing something which may be good for you? How often do you succumb to this disgust and fail to do the task? The answer will tell you.

Let's try a little experiment. Think of something you really want; a drink, a cigarette, your favorite food, a new car.

Now rate it on a scale from 1 to 10 based on these questions: *"How much do I want it? How disappointed will I be if I don't get it? Do I want it, or do I need it, do I really have to have it?"*

Consider how pained you will be if you don't do or get what you're considering. Rate on the scale the statements, *"I have to have a cigarette. I didn't have one yesterday and it ruined my day. I haven't had one for two days, maybe I can wait until tomorrow."*

Once again, we see that the tried-and-true techniques we've used before will work perfectly here. Establishing self-discipline is, after all, a large task which you'll want to break up into smaller tasks, each with a timeline. You'll want to log your activities and progress, state your intentions and get a support partner and so on. Focus, persistence, organization, resilience, responsibility, and a strong work ethic are all traits of people who practice self-discipline.

Self-discipline, like those other traits, are learned behaviors and they are forged in time and experience. And it has its own inherent challenges. If you know these challenges, you'll be better equipped to handle them when they come along.

The road to self-discipline will challenge your perceptions, for instance. It's the old bugaboo of self-efficacy. Some people just don't believe that they can be more disciplined. They are who they are. We've seen this pop in several different ways throughout our studies so far. But it may be particularly challenging when it comes to self-discipline. Why is that? Perhaps because self-discipline goes deeper than almost anything else we've touched on yet. Without self-discipline, all the goal setting and time-logging in the world won't come to much. It may, over time, sharpen one's self-discipline, of course. The methods we discussed are time-tested and laboratory-proven to help defeat procrastination and overthinking, and both of those are rife with a lack of self-discipline. Practicing them will naturally increase your self-discipline as a result.

But what if we turned it around, and put self-discipline where it belongs; as a cause or motivating factor instead of a symptom or a result? We'd see that this is the source of our strengths and our weaknesses. Those who have more self-discipline are better equipped to curb unhealthy behavior, after all.

Some people are lucky enough to have been raised in a strictly regulated home. I don't mean an abusive home, but it's known that children brought up under less supervision and less parental guidance get into more trouble. Kids with a more stable home fare better. Kids who play team sports are recorded as being more prosperous as adults. Why? Discipline is instilled in you in a more stable household or on a sports team.

But not everybody had that kind of upbringing. Some had working parents and were so-called *latch-key* kids. Some kids were loners and not athletic. I was in both categories. And a lot of people who weren't strictly disciplined as kids simply lack self-discipline as adults.

Those who have some self-discipline can always have more, and those who have less need more. Those who have none truly need it. The good news is that it can be learned, and at any time of life.

Some people may tell you that the first seven years of life are the formative years, where the basics of the individual are set. And to a degree, that's probably right. But people don't stop growing at seven years old. They evolve and change and become better people with greater depth. So, it's a fallacy to say that a person has no control over their self-discipline as a result of childhood experiences. It's entirely a personal choice.

So, how do you nurture self-motivation? Really, it brings us back to the set of skills we apply to just about everything. Find your motivation, set your goals, do a time log, get support, delegate if possible, abandon the mental stumbling blocks, practice self-sympathy.

Another way of getting around the challenges of self-discipline is to find a motivational activity. Think of this as the reward you'll get at the end of every small task. This time let it be something like watching an episode of your favorite TV show uninterrupted, or a long, hot bath.

An interesting thing about the quest for self-discipline, as with the other pursuits which should follow it and come before, is that you must become comfortable with failure. Perfectionism is a central challenge of procrastination and overthinking, but those are fueled by self-discipline. If perfectionism infects you at that root level, you may never get anywhere. In your quest for self-discipline, you'll fail several times, perhaps quite often. That's to be expected. Don't let the perfect be the enemy of the good. A fifty-percent success rate, and that's a failure for every success, is awesome. It will increase your self-discipline considerably. If you succeed only three times out of then, you'll hit 50% the next year, and incrementally increase year after year. Accept failure as a necessary part of the process.

HERE ARE A FEW TIPS AND TRICKS TO DEVELOP YOUR SELF-DISCIPLINE:

- Make it a habit by doing it once a day. Pick one thing to deny yourself, to press yourself to do. Just one thing a day, you can do it again the next day if you like, but deny yourself something else. It might be a treat, it might be a margin of tardiness, it might be leaving mail unopened. Sacrifice one of these every day. Not only will you strengthen your self-discipline, you'll actually be getting things done.

- Focus on one facet of your self-discipline at a time. This is a manner of breaking the big task into little tasks, like the previous exercise. But this will also keep you focused on that particular discipline. Distractions and multi-tasking will be especially detrimental here. This week, you'll get the place thoroughly cleaned. Next week, you can organize. The week after that, start getting into shape. You'll never be able to get all that done at once.

- Meditate for 10 minutes a day. We've already taken a brief look at the benefits and practices of meditation. And as it is its own kind of self-discipline and focus, it can only strengthen your self-discipline overall. The mutual benefit is that being more self-disciplined, you'll only get more out of your meditation.

- Here's another exercise to make you more self-disciplined. Make your bed. I know, some of you are balking in one direction or the other. Some people always do it, some people never do. For those who don't, consider the benefits. First, you've accomplished a small task, very first thing in the morning. That's good for self-efficacy. It puts you in a productive mindset. And as we've discussed, the environment mirrors the psyche. A messy bed makes for a messy mind, even if you're not there. Also, you never know who may come home with you, and you don't want to look like a slob.

- While you should have a healthy diet and lifestyle, don't neglect natural sugar intake. We know how too much or too little glucose can affect the brain. Glucose, you'll recall, carries energy to the brain and other organs, muscles, and bodily systems. When you're low on blood sugar, you risk losing motivation. But remember, everything in moderation!

Upon analysis, self-discipline seems rooted in three basic instincts: Self-preservation, self-assertion, and self-fulfillment.

1. Self-preservation takes focus off unimportant things and redirects it toward what is necessary, what is vital for survival. Those with this instinct tend not over overemphasize material goods and tend not to exploit others.
2. Those with a strong sense of self-assertion know what their value is but they're open to letting others speak as well. They're firm but gentle and resist abusive language or treatment of others.
3. Those who have or seek self-fulfillment are also resilient. Self-control urges this person on to facing challenges and

developing the skills necessary for success and happiness; in other words, self-fulfillment.

And these challenging but possibly necessary skills may include things like learning to dance or draw or any artistic pursuit which may take years to do well. These are the ultimate tests of self-discipline. Nobody's going to put that guitar in your hands and a gun to your head, after all ... you hope. That'd be pretty weird.

Self-control makes for a life of happy moderation, not living in the past or the future, neither wanting to much or failing to see when you've had enough.

DEVELOP THE SYSTEM TO BECOME A PRODUCTIVITY HERO!

There are a few modern systems that will help you get things done. We've leaned hard on the Pomodoro method, so let's take a look at a few more.

The *Getting Things Done* (GTD) starts with writing down anything and everything which needs to get done. We've done this before, but we'll rate them a bit differently. Classify them into six categories; current actions, current projects, areas of responsibility, 1-to-2-year goals. 3-to-5-year goals, and life goals.

Do the little ones first, get them out of the way and build up your self-efficacy and build up some momentum. As you might assume by now, break up the bigger projects into smaller milestones. Then proceed as we've done. It's the classifications which matter here. It's a good way to get control of short- and long-term goals. It's a little more advanced than doing a single project this way, but will put you in greater control of your life.

The *Zen to Done* (ZTD) approach is comparable to the Getting Things Done approach, but the Zen approach focuses on habits while the other focuses on the system. ZTD centers on the process, on the doing, in other words, while GTD focuses on creating a system and letting the system do the work.

GTD is a loosely structured timetable for task accomplishment. ZTD structures the day around three most important tasks and the week around major tasks. There's no five-year increment in the ZTD framework. ZTD uses simplification to focus you on essentials, more specific goals in tighter timelines.

ZTD's focus on our habits is central, and there are habits every ZTD master seems to evince. They capture ideas, notes, and tasks so they're not forgotten. They make quick decisions and don't procrastinate. They set most important tasks for each day. They do one task at a time without distractions, no multi-tasking. They keep simple lists and check them daily. They have organized environments with a place for everything. They review their goals and systems regularly and reduce them to which are essential. They set and keep routines and they work passionately at work for which they are passionate.

Sound familiar? Everything we've been working on leads us to this, prepares us for it, makes it not only possible but almost simplistic!

The system known as *Don't Break the Chain* was apparently inspired by comedian Jerry Seinfeld. Not surprisingly, it focuses on creative success. The story goes that the comic bought a calendar and drew a thick red X through every day in which he wrote new material. The idea was that if he didn't write any new material on a given day, he would break the chain of X marks. It may sound simplistic, but it uses almost all the techniques we've discussed in one easy-to-use system. It's a time-log, it's accountability, it's visualizing, it's motivational. X out every day that you do something to accomplish your goal and don't break the chain.

And what is it with airline food, am I right?

You can modify the system though. If you're on vacation, use blue instead of red. Vacationing is part of refreshing your productive cycle, after all. And an X is still an X. But keep it red as much as you can! You can also allow yourself a few gaps in a month, but not two in a row, and not more than one per week. Then hang that calendar in a prominent place, where you can see it, be reminded by it, be inspired by it.

This method won't be great for complex time management or Pomodoro-style milestone projects, just a continued advance toward a single thing. This one is great for self-discipline, because you do that in so many different ways every day, and they're all steps on a single journey. You might also keep several calendars, one for self-discipline, one for personal projects, one for professional projects. You can use the same color-coding system for each to keep them easy to follow.

The *Daily Trifecta* method focuses on three things per day so that those tasks are all completed by the end of the day. It's a good method for short-term goals and for any Pomodoro-style construct.

The *MOSCOW* method breaks up tasks into four categories of differing value: Must-have (M), should have (S), could have (C), and would have (W). Ranking your tasks this way will help you prioritize them, organize them, and then get them done!

Whichever one you choose, the method of choice should be friction-free, adaptable to your personal needs, be easy to learn, encourage working with others, and compatible with other systems. All of the above fit the bill perfectly. Try one, or try a few of them. Combine them as they might serve you best.

Now let's take a closer look at applying these systems to any and every aspect of your life!

IV

REACHING YOUR
UNLIMITED POTENTIAL

HANDLING THE DIFFERENT AREAS OF YOUR LIFE

DROP THE FIXED MINDSET AND START DEVELOPING A GROWTH MINDSET

There's no single way to reach your unlimited potential, of course. There's no magic key. But, like any big task, you can use the set of skills you've already been developing to achieve this daunting task. And it'll be an ongoing task. As it is with self-discipline, it's a constant forge, and you'll either be constantly improving it or risking it backsliding and yourself along with it.

Let's start this section, about reaching your unlimited potential by breaking the big task down to smaller tasks. It works every time.

Perhaps the first milestone for this project will be to look at where potential lies, and that's in the mind. Your thoughts are central to the direction your life will take; we've seen that in a number of ways. Lack of self-efficacy, negative self-talk, and a variety of other unhealthy mental habits stem from your brain, which we've already taken a look at. But what about the actual thoughts? We've looked at the different types of memory, the different ways emotion affects thought. Now let's dig deeper into that influence, and how you can put it all together and start applying it for even more concrete results (if you've been applying these practices and exercises, my guess is that you've already seen a few, even small ones).

So, onward to thoughts. Thoughts can be constructive or destructive to your self-improvement, as we've seen. But thoughts don't exist in a vacuum, they're generated by a mindset. To understand your thoughts and their effects on your behavior and your life, you have to go deeper still, into the complexities of the mindset.

There are basically two mindsets; a *growth* or a *fixed* mindset. Their nature is intuitive. A growth mindset believes a set of skills or even a situation can be changed, improved, that a thing can *grow*. A fixed mindset generally sees things as static, unchangeable, inevitable, that a thing is *fixed*.

Not surprisingly, those with a fixed mindset tend to be depressed and tend toward failure. Those with a growth mindset tend toward satisfaction and success. The good news is that you (or anyone) can change their mindset and thereby change your thought process, going on to change your life.

Qualities like willpower, courage, creativity, diligence, and good communication skills are learned, not innate, as we've seen. Those with a growth mindset are better prepared and more likely to embrace this and to excel at those qualities.

Those with a fixed mindset tend to avoid challenges, give up easily, perceive effort as worthless or a waste of time. They tend to ignore feedback and are threatened by the success of others.

In contrast, those with a growth mindset embrace challenges, they even look forward to them. They persist when challenged, they don't give up easily. They tend to see effort as the path to mastery. They learn from criticism and believe lessons are inspirational and will lead to success.

In one study of 128 children 10 to 11 years of age, two groups were given identical math problems to solve. One group was encouraged with, "You're doing very well. You must be smart!" In the other group, they encouraged with, "You're doing well. You must be trying hard!" The test went on a few more steps, and the final results were clear. The children encouraged for their innate intelligence fared less well than those praised for the growth mindset of trying hard.

Researchers believe this is so because those who's believe in their own intelligence didn't feel they had to try as hard, and so they did less well. Those praised for their attempts responded to that praise by trying even harder, and thus they did better.

You might recognize the connection to the mindsets of optimism and pessimism. And those mindsets are also not innate and can be changed with self-discipline and knowledge. This is important as it relates to our failures; whether we think we can learn from them or merely be defeated by them, for example.

People with a growth mindset tend to bounce back from failure, as we've seen, and they generally come back stronger. They learn from their failures. In fact, the old saying goes something like, *"You learn more from your failures than your successes."* That is a growth mindset in a nutshell. People with fixed mindsets seem to believe that nothing can be learned from success at all. Growth minded people believe that failure leads to success, but those with a fixed mindset tend to see one failure as proof of a pattern of failure, one which cannot be reversed.

Changing this one link in the chain can be invaluable, even crucial, to your personal growth. At the moment of failure, deliberately choose to adopt a growth mindset, even if you never had one before. Force yourself to be an optimist, no matter how difficult or futile that may seem. It's well within anybody's ability to control their mindset, their thoughts, their behaviors, their goals, their achievements, their lives. They just have to see it that way. Hopefully, *you* do.

But these mindsets are related to still one more phenomenon; the self-fulfilling prophecy.

Famed automaker and American titan Henry Ford once said, "Whether you think you can, or you think you can't ... you're right." Research bears this out. People tend to fall victim to the limits they impose upon themselves. If a person believes themselves to be a perpetual loser, they are not likely to have many successes. They will self-sabotage their efforts in the variety of ways we've already looked at. The belief becomes reality, and a self-fulfilling prophecy is fulfilled.

But I'll bet you've already figured that the reverse is also true. The growth-minded person tells themselves that failure can be surmounted, that they are successes at their core. These people are more willing to take chances and reap the benefits of accomplishing new and challenging tasks.

So, know what your general mindset is. Make a few lists, rank the things in your life which you have accomplished, gave up on accomplishing, or still hope to accomplish. Which list is longer, which is shorter? If you have a long list of things you gave up but a short list of things you have to accomplish, you'll know that reflects a fixed mindset, and that's been limiting you.

Once you change your mindset for the better, your whole life will change for the better!

And, like the other mindsets, be diligent! A person can change their mindset deliberately, from fixed to growth, but it can also work the other way. A person with a growth mindset may be dissuaded through years of failure and fall into a fixed mindset if they're not diligent, maintaining self-discipline. Support partners can be essential tools in this case (as in so many of the things we've discussed in this book).

New neuroscientific advances now show that the brain is more flexible than previously thought. Neurons can change over time under the influence of experience. New connections can grow, and old connections can be strengthened. The insulation which speeds up transmission of impulses can be restored or built up! Furthermore, we can influence this growth with concrete actions, things anybody can do, and a lot of them are right in this book: Better nutrition and sleep habits, employing sound strategies, asking the right questions and setting the right goals, practicing heathy habits like reading or playing a musical instrument.

As you can see, changing your mindset to a growth-oriented perspective can actually improve your brain function, and that in turn will help everything else you think and do. This positive cycle feeds itself and an upward spiral is accelerated.

DON'T DISMISS YOUR FEELINGS, YOUR TOPMOST PRIORITY IS YOURSELF

Making yourself a top priority means employing a variety of the techniques you've already used. But it's important to be deliberate about applying them to every facet of your daily life. And since we're harder on ourselves than on others the area of self-care is of vital importance. Add to that the incredible stress in our daily lives, the processed food, the economic demands, the overwhelming amounts of information that pour into our brains, self-care is both the first thing people forget and the last thing they can afford to forgo.

Healthy sleep habits, better diet, daily exercise, self-discipline, the Pomodoro technique, all are great ways to self-care. Abandon perfectionism, practice self-sympathy. Avoid negative self-talk and overthinking. Learn a new skill.

Self-care for students is also especially important. Their schedules are often packed with scholastic, extra-scholastic, and lots of recreational activity. They work hard and they play hard, draining their resources at every turn. Additionally, students seem more prone to procrastination and overthinking than other groups taken as a whole.

But experts recommend other tips and tricks specifically for self-care.

Just say *no*. We've touched on it briefly before, but bears repeating here. Our lives are so filled with people who need us for one thing or another, we're pressured to over-perform. And it's true that a positive mindset is apt to take advantage of opportunities which come along, it's important to be selective, have discretion. You won't have enough time or resources to do everything you're asked to do in life. That will reduce your ability to do things you're already committed to. We've looked at making lists and prioritizing, and you should employ that technique here. Remember that tasks may be urgent or important, both urgent and important, urgent but not important, important but not urgent, and neither urgent nor important. So, dedicate yourself to the things which are important and urgent first. Because of its effects on your long-term goals and because of its effect on your immediate performance, self-care is both important and urgent.

We haven't talked much about taking vacations, though they are excellent rewards to encourage the completion of a big task. Here, it's an even more vital concept. Self-care trips are really powerful ways to maintain your physical and mental wellbeing. Think about spending the weekend at a hot springs resort or a spa, where you can dedicate yourself entirely to self-care, body, and mind. Camping, golf trips, meditation retreats, there is all manner of self-care destinations you might consider. You may also think about a trip to see family (though that might not reduce your stress at all).

Emotional support pets are very popular, and for good reason. They have a calming, soothing influence. They're a little bit of nature right there in the house with you. They can be sounding boards and sources of support. They're loving. Taking care of a pet is in itself a huge task which you break down into smaller tasks of upkeep and interaction. Just the act of having and maintaining a pet will help you defeat procrastination and overthinking, in fact. Go back and take a look, reread a few things with pet ownership in mind, you'll see what I mean.

It really doesn't matter what kind of animal it is. Whatever appeals to you. Some people just love to stroke the fur of a dog or cat or bunny rabbit. Others find solace in the colors and languid motion of exotic fish; others adore their pet birds. Teaching a parrot to talk is a classic example of the Pomodoro technique and will in itself serve just about every practice we've analyzed.

Being organized is especially important to self-care, because being disorganized is the source of such constant stress and confusion in our daily lives. Self-care is hardly doable without being reasonably well-organized.

Cooking at home is an amazing self-care technique. Not only will the food be as pure and natural as you make it, and it will taste better, but you have the benefit of doing the cooking. Cooking incorporates so much of what we've looked at, combining virtually every technique. When you cook, you're learning a new skill, that's good for the brain. Your self-efficacy and positive thought process are escalated. Small tasks are rewarded with deliciousness, plus the pride of accomplishments. It reduces perfectionism but motivates organization and effort and self-sympathy. It's healthier, and it can have a meditative effect. It's a lot more economical too, which not only reduces the related stress but gives you a sense of control over the economy.

Remember to schedule time for self-care every day. Don't break the chain on this one, it's too important.

Self-care is crucially important to those in recovery from or managing a serious illness. Be it recovery from an accident or dealing with a sudden or chronic illness, self-care is at the heart of any recovery regiment. And there are specific things you might think about if you're employing self-care for this purpose.

Interestingly, facing a medical crisis is very much the kind of big tasks we've been looking at throughout this book, the kind of task you've been training for. It employs almost all the things we've discussed, from a growth mindset to the Pomodoro technique. Recovering from a broken leg requires successfully completing a series of milestones; learning to use crutches, getting out of the cast, physical therapy. Recovery from cancer means surgery or radiation, perhaps rounds of chemotherapy; each of them are a milestone to be completed toward the ultimate goal of recovery. There are lots of other now-familiar techniques which are employed (better sleep and diet, more exercise, meditation, self-sympathy, positive thinking, visualizing).

But let's take a closer look at a few concrete ways to self-care if you're facing a significant recovery process.

First off, you'll definitely want to focus on your strengths and on solving problems. Abandon the past and focus on the future. It's true that we've emphasized living in the present and abandoning the past or the future as a way to beat overthinking. But remember too that the future is a great motivator, and it's key to assembling our long-term plans. In this case, lean on the future to get you through the present.

You'll also want to stay focused on your life. Take the focus away from your disease. This won't be easy. You'll need all your self-discipline to resist being obsessed with it; a life-threatening disease, sure, but even a broken leg can dominate every second of your waking thought. It itches under the cast, your football days are over, it may hurt every time it rains or be a constant pain your whole life. There's a lot to worry about.

But draw on the skills you learned in mediation. And remember habits, and how it's better to replace one with its opposite. Replace your focus on the disease or injury with your focus on a loved one, visualize a dream of future success or happiness. Focus on that one thing, at first for five minutes a day, then ten, and so on. Remove distraction and clutter. Anyone can do it.

People facing recovery should pay particular attention to hygiene. Slipping hygiene can be a sign of helplessness, depression, giving up. See friends too, as increasing isolation indicate the same things.

Do one thing you enjoy every day, something for pure pleasure. Watch an episode of your favorite TV show, take a hot bath.

One thing which is often overlooked in the realm of self-care, be it from injury or illness or just of the basic, general variety of self-care.

Clothes.

Clothes are ubiquitous in our society. They signal our status, our priorities, they express who we are. They are like an environment which we carry around everywhere we go. It mirrors our psyche.

If self-care is your aim (or whatever your aim, really) you should take a look at what you're wearing and what you *should* be wearing.

Clothes can either serve to make you more confident (on the job or on a date) or more relaxed (at home after work, on vacation). Dress for the occasion! It's a lot easier to be comfortable in a bathrobe at home, but a lot more difficult to be confident in one at the office.

Clothes reflect who you are and can affect the way you feel about yourself. They can also affect the way others feel about you. Clothing is a vital connection to others and to the world at large.

Clothes are also a good motivator to socialize a bit more. Imagine being all dressed up with nowhere to go.

Also, changing from work clothes to your personal clothes helps you maintain boundaries. You want to prevent your work life from dominating your personal life. Time off is a big part of self-care, after all.

Work shorter hours if you can. In this competitive society, the 8-hour workday is increasingly rare. But to work much more than that causes lack of focus, burnout, a less-impressive result, and that contributes to a downward spiral. But this can happen without us even knowing it. Outside of a workplace setting, in the new gig economy, it's easier and even more necessary to work longer hours. And in the office, workers often stay late or come in early or even forego lunch to get things done. But as we've seen, these overachievers can easily become underachievers, in this case from sheer burnout. Too many hours at the desk leads to all kinds of physical maladies, from knee and back problems to eye strain and circulatory issues, it's physically dangerous. Work shorter hours if you can and get up and walk around a bit every hour or so to prevent blood clots.

To this end, a lot of people now work at stand-up desks. There are a variety of models, all of them easily adjustable for sitting or standing. It's apparently great for posture, overall comfort, productivity and stamina. Hey, Ernest Hemingway wrote standing up, and we all remember him.

But to get back to working shorter hours, standing up or not, consider scheduling fewer hours to get the job done, that will motivate you to spend less time working. A lot of people believe 35 hours should be the max. I personally work about 70 hours a week.

To make the most out of fewer work hours, let's take a look at a few time-tested rules for corporate time management as it relates to holding meetings.

TIME MANAGEMENT FOR THE CORPORATE WORLD

A way to deal with your own struggles with a busy schedule is to have *theme* days. By that, I mean each day might be set aside for a certain type of activity. You might focus on organization on Mondays, scheduling on Tuesdays, personal interaction on Wednesdays, phone calls on Thursdays, organizing the next week's plans on Friday.

But meetings are by far one of the hardest things to manage in the corporate world. There are different personalities with different tasks and different abilities. Meetings tend to go long and that derails careful time planning. Estimates are that workers spend about 15% of their workweek in meetings. Here are some brilliant ways to keep your meetings running smoothly, efficiently, and quickly.

Keep your meetings to five–minutes. The so-called *five-minute rule* illustrates that most people can get their point across in about half a minute. Six people can report their progress and digest their next moves in that time. If five minutes is too few, make it the minimum and ten minutes the max, maybe fifteen. Nothing more than that. The five-minute rule is golden to the efficient corporate manager.

No meeting should go longer than an hour. No meeting has that many people making that many points.

Set one day aside as a *no meetings* day. Wednesday is good, as everybody should be embroiled in the tasks they were set on Monday. They'll be reporting on Thursday and Friday anyway, so why not give them and yourself a break and let you all knuckle down and get the work done? This will also break up the drudgery of the workweek.

End early if you can. Schedule an hour but shoot to wind up at the 50-minute mark. It sets an example for the others to beat their deadlines too. And it gives them an extra ten minutes to get out of meeting mode and back into work mode. It gives you ten extra minutes too, for some quick meditation or to allow for unexpected complexities which may come up.

Don't start your meetings on the hour. It sounds counterintuitive, but it's true. Standard meeting times lull employees into a state of complacency and they can easily wind up coming in late. Making your meeting at 8:19 am sharp will make the meeting seem more important and less routine. It will challenge your employees to be detail oriented, and to show up on time. And if it's a midday meeting, some of your employees may legitimately be running late due to ongoing business. The off-hour meeting time allows them a margin without actually being late.

The *three-bounce rule* is known to most good managers. It states that as soon as a single topic has had three exchanges back-and-forth, the subject is tabled for another meeting. This prevents the subject from dominating the meeting and derailing the other important subjects. It's the cousin to the five-minute rule.

Don't neglect impact; the impact of one person's work has on the team, for good or ill. Every action has an equal and opposite reaction, after all. Actions have consequences, make sure your team members know that.

Always have an agenda. This will keep your meetings running smoothly and on time and prevent anything from getting lost or forgotten. An agenda will tell you how much time you have to spend on each subject. Time it out, in fact. You've got an hour for the meeting and five subjects? None get more than twenty-minutes. Make sure that allows time for unexpected interruptions.

Speaking of interruptions, smartphones are a big distraction throughout the day, so consider making a rule that smartphones are not allowed in meetings.

Employees generally maintain either a *makers* schedule or a *managers* schedule. Managers are used to taking meetings, but makers are used to working more and meeting less, if at all. For a maker, a midday schedule can punch a hole in their productive day, seriously interrupting the workflow and reducing productivity. Managers do little but take meetings. So, if you're scheduling a meeting with a maker, do it first thing in the morning so they can get back to their logo design or writing project. Your managers should be at your disposal just about any time.

All this being said, some meetings should be longer. Your staff will appreciate the perfunctory, efficient meetings, yes. But they also long to reconnect on a certain human level, and the big meetings allow for that. Give them a chance to gossip a little, catch up how the other's wives or husbands or children are doing. Let them be personal in the work context. But do this only when it seems reasonable, not with every little meeting. And when you do let them indulge (and indulge yourself too) keep it from going too long. Ten minutes or so should do it. Then, it's back to work!

Speaking of distractions like Smartphones, there are other common external office distractions you're going to have to keep an eye on, as much as you can. Internal distractions include fatigue, illness, personal problems or concerns, and daydreaming. There's little you can do here but gently support your team member and encourage them to get whatever professional help they need. That's good for them and it's good for your business.

Distractions in the workplace make for between 70% to an astonishing 99% of office employees report feeling distracted. The average employee is distracted roughly 56 times a day. The same studies also tell us that the average worker takes roughly 2 hours over the course of the day transitioning between distractions and actual work.

Distractions take their toll on the workers too. Of those surveyed, 54% of corporate makers or managers report that they feel that they're not performing as well as they should while 50% report being significantly less productive. A full 20% report being unable to reach their full career potential. Greater distractions have been shown to have a negative effect on memory, too.

Mobile phone use, the internet, and gossip are the three leading causes, though not the only ones. Of course, people go on their mobile phones largely to use the internet, so that particular distraction is particularly troublesome.

The internet is a huge distraction, but it's a big part of the workday for so many managers and makers, it's impossible to ban them; ditto, smartphones. But there are apps you can install in your office computers, such as *Strict Workflow* and *StayFocusd*, can limit your workers' access to certain, more distracting websites.

Another common distraction is chatty coworkers. Certainly, you want them to be friendly and to interact freely, but the focus inevitably turns to personal subjects and gossip. This can lead to rumors, feuds, toxic feelings which can become contagious and spread throughout your team. It's best to limit this if you can. But don't be overly authoritarian either. Correct them if you need to, and then be firm and reasonable. Explain that you'd like to get the most out of their efforts during work hours, and other things can be discussed outside work hours, if they must be. And always discourage rumors and gossip. That is never acceptable behavior, especially not in an office setting. It's tempting, and it's fun, but remind them of the benefits of self-discipline and the drawbacks of negativity. Even if they don't agree, my guess is that they'd take the hint.

Avoid office politics too. Make it clear to all that you run a meritocracy. Praise and reward go to those who perform based on results, not based on the person. Sounds familiar, right? Good.

An offshoot of this is the background noise generated by workers who are too loud. Whether they're on the phone with a client or chatting with a coworker, the sheer volume of these voices can become a distraction. It's a more common complaint than you might think among corporate workers today. Try to keep a library rule in the office and limit any chat to a low volume, a short time limit, and a high-value priority. If it's important, make it quick and keep it quiet. Loud eating is a similar annoyance.

Limit personal visits to the office; spouses with children or even pets are very disruptive to the office workflow. You can still have office birthday parties and corporate picnics where everybody is welcome. But office time is for office business.

It's a lot to look after, but I think you'll find it's worthwhile. Studies show that 75% of workers report getting more done with fewer distractions, and 57% of people report feeling motivated to do their very best. Fifty-one percent reported feeling more confident, and 44%

believe their work is improved. Those are impressive numbers but think of all that productivity you're losing if you're not managing your office distractions efficiently.

More practical tips for dealing with distractions include noise-cancelling headphones, which also combats another big distraction; loud coworkers.

We've talked about distractions at work and how to deal with them, but more and more of us work from home, and that's not likely to change. So how do we deal with the distractions of home while doing the work of the office?

Family will have constant demands on you, and of all the people it's hardest to say *no* to, it's your beloved spouse and adorable rug-rats. But you're going to have to be firm, set them all down, and explain that you've got a workday, 8 am to 5 pm or whatever it is. During that time, you are not to be disturbed. Maybe now you're seeing how important it is to train yourself to be able to say *no*, because this will be the greatest test. And it won't just happen once, you may have to remind them from time to time … throughout the day.

Same goes for your neighbors. Your jolly neighbor may spot you at home and assume you've got time for a chat. Kindly correct him. Hey, if you could say no to your family, you can probably disappoint Stanley and Ida next store or across the street.

You might consider inviting your neighbors to enjoy a barbeque to make up for how much time you spent working. That'll have all the benefits of cooking, socializing, and recreating.

Housework is another distraction that's more particular to the home. Offices are generally cleaned by a crew in the middle of the night. But avoid housework as a distraction. Hopefully you have a support partner in your family who can fill the breach. Even your kids may be willing to chip in and help. That would be a good lesson for them in almost everything we've looked at in this book, from self-discipline to self-efficacy to a sense of connection between themselves and their environment.

Food and drink are other home-oriented distractions. You may have a snack machine or a soda machine in the break room, but you probably don't have a fridge full of yummy leftovers, a variety of beverages, hot tea filling the air. Your senses are hard to beat, and they will motivate you to be distracted. Don't be. Hey, nothing worthwhile is ever easy, right? If you backslide here, you'll get less done and put on extra weight, itself the source of all kinds of bad behaviors. Don't say you weren't warned!

MAKING MONEY IS SOMETHING THAT YOU SHOULD ENJOY DOING

Let's be honest. Business is about profit. That profit should not come from the suffering of others, sacrifices and rewards should be evenly distributed. But in the end, business makes money, or they fail. And good corporate management means ensuring the company's success, not its failure. The corporate success is your big long-term task, everything else you do professionally is a milestone. Some of those are so big they're their own big tasks, which are broken down, and so forth.

But money carries baggage for a lot of people. They may have feelings of guilt over having too much or shame over having too little. It changes some and can ruin others. Yet it's something we absolutely need. And it's part of the cycle of positive behavior. Money means success, freedom to enjoy the finer things in life. It allows us to help those in want or need. It allows us to extricate ourselves from emergencies, bringing stability and a lack of stress. As much as we hate to admit it, it's what a lot of us are working so hard for.

There are basically two direction money flows, in and out. It may come in as income, dividends or investment profits, inheritance, fluke things like lottery wins. It goes out in the form of expenses like food and shelter, transportation and necessities, luxuries and amusement, taxes and loan penalties.

Investments and savings represent a strange dichotomy. The cash may move out of your bank account, but it moves into your stock portfolio, so it isn't really spent. But it's still not in your bank account either. Savings, on the other hand, represents money that moves in and doesn't move out. Savings are harder to come by these days, and it's a crucial part of financial stability. Most Americans asked today report having less than $400 dollars in the bank.

If you're finances are slipping out of your control, always fall back on what you've learned here. If paying off a credit card is a big task, break it up Pomodoro style, and tackle it in smaller chunks (as long as they meet the minimum monthly payment, of course).

The first thing to do to tackle your personal finances, you may not be surprised to hear, is to make a series of lists, logs, and plans. The first thing you need is a budget. Write down how much you earn in a month and add it up, then how much you spend; on necessities like rent and food, and on luxuries. If your luxury column is too high, simply reduce spending on those things. Sacrifice them until your finances are back on track. Then you can return to one or two of them, if you still want to.

Common luxuries you can surely cut off the list (temporarily) is eating out. Homemade food tastes better than prepared food, and you get all the benefits of cooking; the meditative and creative and organizational skills, the instant gratification, the boom in self-confidence.

Allocate about 20% of your income to financial priorities, and 30% toward lifestyle spending. But stick to that and don't let the thirty become thirty-five, forty, or even more. Since your rent or mortgage is probably about 30% of your income, your personal spending should be necessarily limited.

Cut those credit card bills by paying a certain amount over the minimum every month. Otherwise you'll never get out from under them. While you're at it, cut cable. You're paying a lot for things you don't watch. Why not skip and watch just what you want on YouTube? At least you can skip the ad in 5 ... 4 ... 3 ... 2 ...

You may want to put the cards away for a while. Don't make a bad situation worse. Commit to going to a cash-only basis for one week a month. Stay away from those credit cards!

Plan to put something away for savings every month. Make it the same amount every month and make you deposit on the same day every month. You can create a special savings account and then transfer the money online, so a visit to the bank isn't even necessary.

Some people enjoy a spending fast, where they set about to spend nothing for a given period. Can you go two days? Three? Five? Even if you can't do more than two, you're still saving.

Don't commit to any recurring monthly charges. You can lose track and wind up spending monthly on things you don't need or perhaps even want. If you have ongoing charges, make a list of them and track them by expense and value. Think about reducing your current ongoing charges by half or more if you can. The savings will add up automatically if you just cut loose that Netflix subscription.

Another good way to watch your finances is good ol'-fashioned bargain hunting. They're around more and more. Smartphone apps are dedicated to saving you money on car insurance, nights out, all manner of items you may be spending too much for. There are also retail outlet stores which offer heavily discounted merchandise. When grocery shopping, always keep an eye out for the sale deals. And take your local supermarket on a savings club card if they have one. You could save up to or more than 20% per visit to the grocery store.

Like a lot of the things we've discussed, being good with money takes practice, but there are lots of good ways to do it. And the results are sure to make your life and your other efforts a lot easier and more stress-free.

Managing money, as much as anything we've discussed, requires a support friend. This person could be your spouse, your business manager, your accountant, a friend, or a family member. But you'll need help somewhere along the line, for sure. This particular long-term task may require more than one friend, but a whole support network. Your spouse and children, if you have them, should be involved in the campaign, helping to save too.

Here are yet a few more handy tricks when it comes to money:

Never cosign a loan. It will corrode a family relationship, and it could destroy your credit and cost you a fortune. This time it should be easy to say *no*. That being said, a lot of parents cosign loans for their newly adult children; first cars, apartment leases. But this is not the usual and even than can be fraught with difficulties.

If you're a student, go after every federal loan or grant or scholarship you can find. Avoid student loans like the plague if you can. If you're already struggling with payments like these, look into federal plans for assistance or other repayment options.

LIVING A LEISURE LIFE ON TOP OF YOUR RESPONSIBILITIES

And all this planning could and should lead you to a bit more free time. But how you spend that free time is important to your overall plan. If you live healthily on the weekdays and then go out and trash yourself on the weekends, you will suffer a reduction of productivity later.

Research indicates that adults in the US enjoy roughly 40 hours of time away from work. Men and women seem to spend about five hours a day in so-called *free time*. This is time outside of the responsibilities of household chores, work, curricular and religious activities. Watching TV, sitting in the hot tub, whatever.

Free time tends to draw us to activities or events, but not all are of equal value. When presented with a free time opportunity, ask yourself, "Will this give me a good story to tell? Will it change me in some positive way? Will it allow me to relax and support my personal relationships? Is it challenging? Does it fill me with a sense of wonder, fill my heart with the milk of human kindness? Does it improve my social standing? Will it bring comfort or happiness to someone I love?"

If the answer is *yes*, you should definitely go. If not, give them stronger consideration and more discretion.

NO MAN IS AN ISLAND, THE RELATIONSHIPS YOU BUILD ARE NECESSARY FOR YOUR LIFE

One of the best ways to strengthen any relationship, is to be a good listener. It's been said that the best conversationalist you'll ever meet only talks about one subject ... you. And this is largely true. First of all, we're a self-centered culture, and very few people do anything but go on and on about themselves anyway. Instead of competing for their attention, which may not be worth having in the first place, just give them what they want. Ask them about themselves, deflect questions about yourself, and be a good listener. It doesn't do much good if you're constantly asking question after question, interrupting the answers you're supposed to be listening to. Just listen.

Still, that's not as easy as it sounds. Our competitive environment encourages us to speak up for ourselves, to toot our own horns, to think the most of ourselves, to make the most of ourselves and every opportunity. But a lot of that means presenting yourself as a caring, interested person, somebody not bent on making the most of every opportunity but allowing the other person to do the same.

It does take surprising will and self-control. And like all the things we've talked about so far, it requires a certain depth of understanding. And there's more to the art of listening than you may know.

First, there will always be some discrepancy between what a person intends to say and how you interpret that. It's a natural drawback of language. And it's made worse by emails and text, which lack all the subtleties and reactive possibilities of a live conversation where you can at least hear the person's voice and see their face. There's no better way to be misunderstood than to send an email or text.

Language is important because it is what best represents us. You can't judge a book by its cover, they say, but a person's language is what is printed on the pages of their soul.

And there are two varieties of the art of listening. There is passive and active listening, and you must know which is best and which you lean toward in order to make the most of your relationship.

The passive listener doesn't really listen, they just tolerate their time to wait until they can deliver their position. They're not about to be swayed or really even engaged. The active listener takes into account what the other is saying, digesting it, ready to be moved by it.

It's impossible to miss the parallel between a growth mindset or a fixed mindset. The passive listener is likely to have a fixed mindset, unwilling to consider the possibilities of change. The active listener, change-oriented, is vastly more likely to be of a growth mindset.

Spending time with friends and family is crucial to strengthen your relationships, for obvious reasons. These are the strongest relationships you have. Your most formative influences were first your family and then your friends, so these are the groups who are best served to be your support network, the cradle of your non-professional life.

Such an intimate support network, as opposed to a work support network of friendly coworkers, offers a sense of belonging, security, increased self-worth. It is said to reduce your stress levels (if you're not in my family!) and all jokes aside, studies bear this out.

Romantic relationships, like familial relationships and longtime friendships, will have highs and lows over the years as the individuals experience their own changes. So, you really should be as willing to be tolerant of the other person's changes, as you would expect that person would do for you, Remember the so-called *Golden Rule: Do unto others as you would have them to unto you.*

Relationships are unique, so each has to be dealt with on its own terms. If you're willing to deal with the other person in your life on their terms, you've got a good chance. If you're only willing to deal on your own terms, you might wind up alone. But your partner will face the same challenges, so think of it as facing them together.

Relationships of all sorts are about two things; feelings and communications. So often, we feel one thing but say another, to protect ourselves or because we lack the skills to say what we truly feel. That's not as easy as it sounds either. For example, you may have respect for a person, but that's not enough if you act out and treat them disrespectfully. You have to show respect, or your feelings are irrelevant to that person. It's not enough to love, you have to show love, communicate it successfully.

The flipside of that coin isn't showing it but receiving that feeling. A person may simply not feel loved or understood. You always have to keep in mind, not only what you are feeling and perhaps failing to communicate, but what the other is hearing and perhaps failing to process.

If you disagree, remain respectful. Don't personalize it. Think of the emphasis on the results of the task or on the value of the worker. The healthier focus is on the thing, not the person. And this only makes sense because a thing cannot be insecure or insulted or lash out, but a person will be more than ready to do so. So be resolved to be as respectful as you can in disagreements. Don't insist on being right but do express yourself so you can avoid overthinking later!

For a successful relationship, don't cut yourself off from other interests and relationships. A happy life is a well-rounded life. The more which enriches you outside the relationship, the more you can bring to the relationship.

And beware of any relationship partner who tries to separate you from your family or your friends, unless they truly are abusive in a criminal sense. The concept of a *splitter,* or a *wedge personality*, is a well-known element in relationships. This is a personality who seeks to isolate and control the other person, destroying their trust in their previous relationships.

Remember that there's a difference between *falling* in love and *staying* in love. The first may be chaotic and random, but the second is almost always the result of a determined effort from both parties.

Otherwise, everything in this book covers romance as if it were a big, long-term goal (a life's love) made up of a series of goals and milestones (dating, engagement, marriage, staying married) which are rewarded and require planning and a positive mindset and so on. Tilt it just the right way, you've just read the best dating manual ever! To touch on just a few, the techniques we've learned which come into play most in the romantic arena include scheduled commitment (weekends, celebrations), learning new skills (which you share, like dance classes or wine tasting), recreation and self-care (and mutual care, in this case), volunteer together (at a food bank or helping with a city cleaning initiative),

Do things together that benefit others. Communicate clearly and respectfully but also take note of the physical cues you may get from the other. And be honest, as your body language is likely to give you away and you don't want to be rightfully called out as a liar.

Beware of stress, which may make you misread what your partner is saying or conveying. In times of stress, it might be best to avoid going too deep. Wait until you're both calmer and more reasonable. Remember the influence of emotion on our behavior and act accordingly.

As with the other things we've looked at, it's crucial to abandon perfectionism in a relationship. Nobody's perfect, and no coupling is absolutely perfect.

A HEARTY SPIRITUAL LIFE

Well, maybe God is perfect, which is one of the most attractive aspects of religion. It not only provides regiment to our lives, and socialization, education, even philosophy. Some focus more on the ethereal aspect, others on the more earthbound social aspect. Either way, it can be very good for developing personal skills and becoming a better, happier, and more well-rounded person.

The benefits of spirituality include reassurance, a clearer view of perfectionism and its faults but at the same time fostering a stronger sense of self-efficacy and value and that encourages positive self-talk. Spirituality can provide meaning, something to focus on in the way of meditation. It helps foster sympathy for others and connections to others, and generates a growth mindset.

Research shows that religious people recovered faster from various types of heart surgery than those of weaker faith or no faith at all! Those who attend religious services seem to live longer than those who don't.

To seek a more spiritually grounded life, any of the major organized religions will give you ample opportunities. There's no time to survey them here, but your libraries, bookstores, and internet outlets are filled with books on all of them, and from every different angle.

Once you find the religion which best expresses your beliefs, participate. Jesus said, "Faith without works is dead." So, get out there and act on that faith. You'll find it has every benefit of the many tips and techniques we've already discussed, and for the same reasons. It's great for positive self-talk, socialization, gratification, focus, stress reduction, and more!

Make sure the organization you join is more spiritual than an organization, if you take my meaning. A church may ask for up to 10% of your income as a tithing, or contribution to the functioning of the church, and most small churches need that. A legitimate organization will encourage you to get closer to your family and friends. Any organization that asks for more than 10% or tries to separate you from your family and friends is to be avoided at all costs.

Become comfortable with the notion of prayer. It's not so different than having a support partner, only that might be the like of Christ Jesus Himself! You've got a sounding board and a mentor.

Reading religious texts has all the benefits of reading anything else. It stimulates the brain, it invigorates the creative spirit, it encourages focus in the face of infinite distraction.

Share your experiences and views with others. Give voice to it and make it real. This is especially potent in the context of the Abrahamic religions, Judaism especially.

Well, we started deep inside ourselves, and we wound up in the heavens themselves. Hopefully, you've learned a lot along the way. If something seems less clear, don't worry. There was a lot to digest. Go back and read it again, just the relevant sections if you like. This book was written for you, so by all means make the most of it!

CONCLUSION

Congratulations! You've just been exposed to the latest and best information about procrastination and overthinking and a good deal more than that. You've got a handful of tips and trick to apply this knowledge to your everyday life. You're now able to adapt a different mindset, a better perspective, with greater understanding of the challenges you and others face in your daily personal and professional lives. You've got everything you need to live a happier, more successful, and more fulfilling life. You've got the tools to correct a downward spiral, to reverse negative self-talk and a fixed mindset. You're ready try meditation, you can see the benefits of a healthier lifestyle. And everything you now know can be applied to your life immediately. Other than a few little materials, you've got everything you need to correct a lifetime of negativity and create the life you've always wanted. One of Albert Einstein's guiding principles was that if you can visualize it, it is possible. Think about that, and start seeing what your future is going to be like once you apply the data, lessons, and techniques you learned in this book.

We started by digging into the deepest center of your core thoughts and beliefs. Then worked outward to virtually every part of your body. We went further, through your clothes and your immediate environment to the people around you, personal, and professional. We looked at the mutual influence we all share, then reached further out to social ramification, to a worldwide pandemic of procrastination and overthinking, the negative self-talk, and limiting mindset which are true for people all over the world. We went to the Far East for remedies like meditation. We transcended Earth and looked to the heavens for support, to India for the wisdom of Buddhism.

And it all comes back to you; your life on every level. You've got what it takes to improve your life and to help others improve their lives. I'd wish you good luck, but you no longer need it. You've already got everything you need to take the next steps toward a brighter future. As I said at the beginning of this book, your life is on the precipice of great change. It's up to you!

9 781801 342247